MOWRY'S
Basic nutrition and
diet therapy

MOWRY'S

Basic nutrition and diet therapy

SUE RODWELL WILLIAMS, R.D., M.R.Ed., M.P.H., Ph.D

Chief, Nutrition Program, Kaiser-Permanente Medical Center,
Oakland, California; Instructor, Nutritional Science and Clinical Nutrition,
Health Sciences Division, Chabot College, Hayward, California;
Field Faculty, M.P.H.–Dietetic Internship Program, and Coordinated
Undergraduate Program in Dietetics, University of California,
Berkeley, California

Illustrated

SIXTH EDITION

The C. V. Mosby Company

ST. LOUIS · TORONTO · LONDON   1980

SIXTH EDITION

Copyright © 1980 by The C. V. Mosby Company

All rights reserved. No part of this book may be reproduced
in any manner without written permission of the publisher.

Previous editions copyrighted 1958, 1962, 1966, 1969, 1975

Printed in the United States of America

The C. V. Mosby Company
11830 Westline Industrial Drive, St. Louis, Missouri 63141

Library of Congress Cataloging in Publication Data

Mowry, Lillian.
    Mowry's Basic nutrition and diet therapy.

    Bibliography: p.
    Includes index.
    1. Diet therapy.   2. Nutrition.   I. Williams, Sue
Rodwell, 1922-   II. Title.   III. Title: Basic
nutrition and diet therapy.
RM216.M64   1980   615'.854   79-26165
ISBN 0-8016-5556-0

C/VH/VH   9   8   7   6   5   4   3   2   1   03/C/328

*To all those whose efforts in the past
have made possible our present knowledge of nutrition
and its role in preserving human health
and in advancing diet therapy*

Preface

Since its first edition over a decade ago, *Mowry's Basic Nutrition and Diet Therapy* (originally published under the title *Nutrition and Diet Therapy for Practical Nurses*) has provided a sound and comprehensive text for practical and licensed vocational nursing programs. Through the years prior to her death, Lillian Mowry, its able author, maintained a high level of quality and purpose through a number of editions, and the book filled a practical need among various paramedical personnel for a realistic and easily comprehended reference. With the preceding edition and in this sixth edition, I have accepted the task of continuing to maintain a worthy basic nutrition text for readers, students, and practitioners in nursing and related health fields.

I have greatly appreciated the many letters from teachers and health workers throughout the United States who are using the text and who have sent helpful evaluations and suggestions. I cherish these communications. I hope you will continue to express to the publishers and to me your experience with the book and your needs. We will do our best to fulfill these needs in subsequent editions.

My basic objective in this edition, as in preceding editions, has been to maintain the book's style, general purpose, and organization, developing current material and references and applying the material to focus on personalized patient care.

For example, in Part one, "Principles of nutrition," the recommended dietary allowances of the Food and Nutrition Board of the National Research Council are presented. These statements of nutrient needs are discussed in terms of their broad implications for human health. Because of the significance of these nutrient needs for optimum health, the standards for their use are integrated with discussions of each of the nutrients themselves. Also, to supplement these nutritional guides and provide a more comprehensive food planning and diet analysis tool, the table of the basic four food groups has been enlarged in terms of food types and quantities and the major nutrient contributions of each group.

Part two, "Community nutrition: the life cycle," a new section in the preceding edition, continues to focus on this increasing area of concern and on health care activities.

Part three, "Diet therapy," applies current basic knowledge in nutritional science to care of patients with clinical disease.

As needs indicate, in future editions I plan to further develop current concepts of nutrition to provide needed perspective and balance in a rapidly expanding and changing scientific and social world. Throughout, my two basic goals will remain: (1) to present current, sound nutrition knowledge and practice in a clear, comprehensive style and (2) to focus on a practical, person-centered approach to meeting the needs of individuals and families.

Thus it is my earnest hope that this book will continue to guide those using it to a clear understanding of some of the elemental principles of nutritional science and to a realistic concern for applying them to human need. To this end I invite and encourage your communication. We share a common purpose.

Sue Rodwell Williams

Contents

PART ONE

PRINCIPLES OF NUTRITION

1

The importance of a balanced diet

Nutrition concerns the food we eat and how our bodies use it. Nutritional science is the study of the scientific laws governing the food requirements of human beings for maintenance, growth, activity, reproduction, and lactation. Good nutrition is essential to good health throughout life, beginning with prenatal life and extending through old age.

Dietetics is the practical application of these laws to persons and groups of persons in various conditions of health and disease.

Food has always been one of the prime necessities of life. Too many people, however, are concerned only with food that relieves their hunger or satisfies their appetites but are not concerned with whether it supplies their bodies with all the components of good nutrition.

The physician, the nurse, and the nutritionist or dietitian are all aware of the important part that food plays in maintaining good health in the normal person and in the recovery of the person who is ill. Chronic ill health in a person cannot be accepted without checking on his food habits as a possible contributing factor. Thus, a primary activity in planning care in any situation is assessing the patient's nutritional status and identifying nutritional needs.

The well-nourished person is much more likely to be alert, both mentally and physically, and to have a happy outlook on life. He is also more able to resist infectious diseases than the undernourished person. Proper diet not only makes him a healthier person but also extends the period of his normal activity for more years.

Food must perform three functions within the body:
1. Provide heat and energy
2. Contain the necessary nutrients to build and repair the tissues of the body
3. Supply the nutrients necessary to regulate the body processes

The nutrients that perform these three functions within the body have sometimes been called "the seven wonders of the world."

3

Carbohydrates ⎫
Fats ⎫ ⎬ Nutrients that produce energy
Proteins ⎬ ⎭
Nutrients that build or repair ⎬ Minerals ⎬
Water ⎭ Nutrients that regulate body
Vitamins processes
Cellulose

Good nutrition, then, means that an individual receives and utilizes substances that are obtained from a diet containing carbohydrates, fats, proteins, certain minerals, vitamins, water, and cellulose in optimum amounts. The optimum amounts of these nutrients should be greater than the minimum requirements to make provision for variations in health and disease and for the accumulation of some reserves. Dietary surveys have shown that approximately one third of the United States population is living on diets below the optimum level. This does not necessarily mean that one third of American people are undernourished. Some persons can maintain good health on somewhat less than the optimum amounts of the various nutrients. On the average, however, a person receiving less than the optimum amounts will have a greater risk of physical illness than a person receiving the proper amounts.

Evidence of good nutrition is a well-developed body, ideal weight for body size, and good muscles. The skin is smooth and clear, the hair is glossy, and the eyes are clear and bright. Posture is good, and the facial expression is alert. The appetite, digestion, and elimination are good. Compare the more detailed evidences of good and poor states of nutrition given in Table 1-1.

The meal patterns that individuals follow vary with living situations and energy demands. Usually the person who eats a nutritionally well-balanced meal at the beginning of the day can work more efficiently and will avoid the midmorning feeling of fatigue.

With our food environment rapidly changing to include more processed food items of variable or unknown nutrient quality, in some ways American dietary habits have deteriorated in the last few years. In the midst of a plentiful food supply, surveys give increasing evidence of malnutrition, even in hospitalized patients.* The appalling report of a national inquiry board† should be read carefully by every concerned American. Nurses and other health workers have a signal responsibility here.

---

*Butterworth, C. E., Jr.: The skeleton in the hospital closet, Nutrition Today 9(2):4-8, March-April, 1974; and Butterworth, C. E., Jr., and Blackburn, G. L.: Hospital malnutrition, Nutrition Today 10(2):8-18, March-April, 1975.
†Hunger, U. S. A., a report by the Citizen's Board of Inquiry into Hunger and Malnutrition in the U.S., Boston, 1968, Beacon Press.

Table 1-1. Clinical signs of nutritional status*

	Good	Poor
General appearance	Alert, responsive	Listless, apathetic; cachexia
Hair	Shiny, lustrous; healthy scalp	Stringy, dull, brittle, dry, depigmented
Neck glands	No enlargement	Thyroid enlarged
Skin, face and neck	Smooth, slightly moist; good color, reddish pink mucous membranes	Greasy, discolored, scaly
Eyes	Bright, clear; no fatigue circles	Dryness, signs of infection, increased vascularity, glassiness, thickened conjunctiva
Lips	Good color, moist	Dry, scaly, swollen; angular lesions (stomatitis)
Tongue	Good pink color, surface papillae present, no lesions	Papillary atrophy, smooth appearance; swollen, red, beefy (glossitis)
Gums	Good pink color, no swelling or bleeding; firm	Marginal redness or swelling; receding, spongy
Teeth	Straight, no crowding; well-shaped jaw; clean, no discoloration	Unfilled caries, absent teeth, worn surfaces, mottled, malpositioned
Skin, general	Smooth, slightly moist, good color	Rough, dry, scaly, pale, pigmented, irritated; petechiae, bruises
Abdomen	Flat	Swollen
Legs, feet	No tenderness, weakness, or swelling; good color	Edema, tender calf; tingling, weakness
Skeleton	No malformations	Bowlegs, knock-knees, chest deformity at diaphragm, beaded ribs, prominent scapulae
Weight	Normal for height, age, body build	Overweight or underweight
Posture	Erect, arms and legs straight, abdomen in, chest out	Sagging shoulders, sunken chest, humped back
Muscles	Well developed, firm	Flaccid, poor tone; undeveloped, tender
Nervous control	Good attention span for age; does not cry easily, not irritable or restless	Inattentive, irritable
Gastrointestinal function	Good appetite and digestion; normal, regular elimination	Anorexia, indigestion, constipation or diarrhea
General vitality	Endurance, energetic, sleeps well at night; vigorous	Easily fatigued, no energy, falls asleep in school, looks tired, apathetic

*From Williams, S. R.: Nutrition and diet therapy, ed. 3, St. Louis, 1977, The C. V. Mosby Co., p. 393.

Table. 1-2. Recommended daily dietary allowances,[a] revised 1979*

	Age (yr.)	Weight kg.	Weight lbs.	Height cm.	Height in.	Protein (gm.)	Fat-soluble vitamins Vitamin A (µg. R.E.)[b]	Vitamin D (µg)[c]	Vitamin E (mg. α T.E.)[d]	Vitamin C (mg.)
Infants	0.0-0.5	6	13	60	24	kg × 2.2	420	10	3	35
	0.5-1.0	9	20	71	28	kg × 2.0	400	10	4	35
Children	1-3	13	29	90	35	23	400	10	5	45
	4-6	20	44	112	44	30	500	10	6	45
	7-10	28	62	132	52	34	700	10	7	45
Males	11-14	45	99	157	62	45	1000	10	8	50
	15-18	66	145	176	69	56	1000	10	10	60
	19-22	70	154	177	70	56	1000	7.5	10	60
	23-50	70	154	178	70	56	1000	5	10	60
	51+	70	154	178	70	56	1000	5	10	60
Females	11-14	46	101	157	62	46	800	10	8	50
	15-18	55	120	163	64	46	800	10	8	60
	19-22	55	120	163	64	44	800	7.5	8	60
	23-50	55	120	163	64	44	800	5	8	60
	51+	55	120	163	64	44	800	5	8	60
Pregnant						+30	+200	+5	+2	+20
Lactating						+20	+400	+5	+3	+40

*From Food and Nutrition Board, National Academy of Sciences–National Research Council: Recommended dietary
[a]The allowances are intended to provide for individual variations among most normal persons as they live in the United
nutrients for which human requirements have been less well defined. See text for detailed discussion of allowances and
average energy intakes.
[b]Retinol equivalents. 1 retinol equivalent = 1 µg. retinol or 6 µg. foarotene. See text for calculation of vitamin A activity
[c]As cholecaliferol. 10 µg. cholecalciferol = 400 I.U. vitamin D.
[d]α tocopherol equivalents. 1 mg. d-α-tocopherol = 1 α T.E. See text for variation in allowances and calculation of vitamin
[e]1 XY (alacin equivalent) is equal to 1 mg. of niacin or 60 mg. of dietary tryptophan.
[f]The folacin allowances refer to dietary sources as determined by *Lactobacillus gases* assay after treatment with enzymes
[g]The FDA for vitamin B_{12} in infants is based on average concentration of the vitamin in human milk. The allowances after
factors such as intestinal absorption; see text.
[h]The increased requirement during pregnancy cannot be met by the iron content of habitual American diets nor by the
during lactation are not substantially different from those of nonpregnant women, but continued supplementation of the

Water-soluble vitamins						Minerals					
Thia-min (mg.)	Ribo-flavin (mg.)	Niacin (mg. M.E.)e	Vita-min B6 (mg.)	Fola-cinf (μg)	Vita-min B12 (μg)	Cal-cium (mg.)	Phos-phorus (mg.)	Mag-nesium (mg.)	Iron (mg.)	Zinc (mg.)	Iodine (μg)
0.3	0.4	6	0.3	30	0.5g	360	240	50	10	3	40
0.5	0.6	8	0.6	45	1.5	540	360	70	15	5	50
0.7	0.8	9	0.9	100	2.0	800	800	150	15	10	70
0.9	1.0	11	1.3	200	2.5	800	800	200	10	10	90
1.2	1.4	16	1.6	300	3.0	800	800	250	10	10	120
1.4	1.6	18	1.8	400	3.0	1200	1200	350	18	15	150
1.4	1.7	18	2.0	400	3.0	1200	1200	400	18	15	150
1.5	1.7	19	2.2	400	3.0	800	800	350	10	15	150
1.4	1.6	18	2.2	400	3.0	800	800	350	10	15	150
1.2	1.4	16	2.2	400	3.0	800	800	350	10	15	150
1.1	1.3	15	1.8	400	3.0	1200	1200	300	18	15	150
1.1	1.3	14	2.0	400	3.0	1200	1200	300	18	15	150
1.1	1.3	14	2.0	400	3.0	800	800	300	18	15	150
1.0	1.2	13	2.0	400	3.0	800	800	300	18	15	150
1.0	1.2	13	2.0	400	3.0	800	800	300	10	15	150
+0.4	+0.3	+2	+0.6	+400	+1.0	+400	+400	+150	h	+5	+25
+0.5	+0.5	+5	+0.5	+100	+1.0	+400	+400	+150	h	+10	+50

allowances, revised 1979, Washington, D.C., 1979, The Academy.
States under usual environmental stresses. Diets should be based on a variety of common foods in order to provide other
of nutrients not tabulated. See Table [B] for weights and heights by individual year of age. See Table [5-3] for suggested

of diets as retinol equivalents.

E activity of the diet as α tocopherol equivalents.

("conjugases") to make polyglutamyl forms of the vitamin available to the test organism.
weaning are based on energy intake (as recommended by the American Academy of Pediatrics) and consideration of other

existing iron stores of many women; therefore the use of 30-60 mg. of supplemental iron is recommended. Iron needs
mother for 2-3 months after parturition is advisable in order to replenish stores depleted by pregnancy.

THE RECOMMENDED DAILY DIETARY ALLOWANCES

In May, 1941, the first meeting of The National Research Council was held in Washington, D. C. This meeting was followed by the publication of the *Recommended Daily Dietary Allowances* by the Food and Nutrition Board of the Council. These recommended allowances are revised about every 5 years to reflect current research findings in nutritional science. The current standards are given in Table 1-2. See also Table 5-3 (p. 28) and Table B (p. 200).

THE BASIC FOUR FOOD GROUPS

The data contained in the recommended allowances (Table 1-2) have been translated into The Basic Four Food Groups (Table 1-3), which provide a general though useful daily food guide for planning meals and evaluating a person's basic food intake pattern.

Additional calories as needed may come from increased servings of the foods listed or from adding food items.

A daily plan consists of three or more meals, each supplying a portion of the day's total food requirement. Following is a sample plan for daily meals:

Breakfast

> *Fruit* rich in vitamin C
> *Cereal* and/or
> *Toast*, roll, or hot bread
> *Butter* or fortified margarine
> *Milk* for cereal and beverage
> *Egg* served frequently (When eggs are not served, include extra milk to give the necessary animal protein.)
> *Coffee* for adults

Lunch

> *Main dish*—should contain eggs, cheese, meat, fish, or poultry (could be soup, salad, sandwich, or a casserole dish)
> *Vegetable*, preferably raw
> *Bread* and *butter* or fortified margarine
> *Simple dessert*, such as custard, gelatin, ice cream, or fruit
> *Milk* for children

Dinner

> *Meat, poultry,* or *fish*, at least 2 oz. per person
> *Vegetables* (two) (one may be potatoes and the other a green leafy or yellow vegetable)
> *Salad*, vegetable or fruit
> *Dessert*—a fruit if a vegetable salad has been used unless fruit was used for dessert at noon
> *Milk* for children

Table 1-3. Daily food guide—The Basic Four Food Groups

Food group	Main nutrients	Daily amounts*
Milk		
Milk, cheese, ice cream, or other products made with whole or skimmed milk	Calcium Protein Riboflavin	Children under 9: 2 to 3 cups Children 9 to 12: 3 or more cups Teenagers: 4 or more cups Adults: 2 or more cups Pregnant women: 3 or more cups Nursing mothers: 4 or more cups (1 cup = 8 oz. fluid milk or designated milk equivalent†)
Meats		
Beef, veal, lamb, pork, poultry, fish, eggs	Protein Iron Thiamine	2 or more servings Count as one serving: 2 to 3 oz. lean, boneless, cooked meat, poultry, or fish
Alternates: dry beans and peas, nuts, peanut butter	Niacin Riboflavin	2 eggs 1 cup cooked dry beans or peas 4 tbs. peanut butter
Vegetables and fruits		4 or more servings Count as 1 serving: ½ cup vegetable or fruit or a portion such as 1 medium apple, banana, orange, potato, or half a medium grapefruit or melon
	Vitamin A	Include: 1 dark green or deep yellow vegetable or fruit rich in vitamin A, at least every other day
	Vitamin C (ascorbic acid) Smaller amounts of other vitamins and minerals	1 citrus or other fruit or vegetable rich in vitamin C daily Other vegetables and fruits, including potatoes
Bread and cereals		4 or more servings of whole-grain, enriched, or restored Count as 1 serving:
	Thiamine Niacin Riboflavin Iron Protein	1 slice bread 1 oz. (1 cup) ready-to-eat cereal, flake or puff varieties ½ to ¾ cup cooked cereal ½ to ¾ cup cooked pasta (macaroni, spaghetti, noodles) Crackers: 5 saltines, 2 squares graham crackers, and so forth

*Use additional amounts of these foods or added butter, margarine, oils, sugars, and so forth, as desired or needed.

†Milk equivalents: 1 oz. cheddar cheese, 3 servings cottage cheese, 1 cup fluid skimmed milk, 1 cup buttermilk, ¼ cup dry skimmed milk powder, 1 cup ice milk, 1⅔ cup ice cream, ½ cup evaporated milk.

FOOD MISINFORMATION

Some persons seem more ready than others to believe false information given out by quacks and health food faddists. These persons may be seeking to preserve youthful vigor, relieve the pain of a chronic illness, or enhance beauty or athletic ability. More effort is now being made by health workers than in the past to teach the public the importance of eating a balanced diet.

The communication of sound nutritional information in a manner that meets individual needs provides the basis for building sound food habits. A real danger in nutritional misinformation, especially for persons with health problems, is that they often postpone obtaining the proper medical attention until it is too late. The American Medical Association has estimated that nutritional quackery costs 10 million Americans several million dollars a year. Sound knowledge of foods and nutrition can help counteract the influence of food faddists.

Questions on the importance of a balanced diet

1. Define nutrition.
2. What is dietetics?
3. What functions must food perform within the body?
4. What nutrients are necessary to provide good nutrition?
5. Why should the optimum required amounts of nutrients be taken?
6. How has the American diet changed in the last few years?
7. Plan a day's menu in accordance with the suggested pattern for daily needs.
8. What are some evidences of good nutrition?
9. Make a list of ways in which you could help to combat food misinformation.
10. What is the approximate cost of food faddism per year to the American people?

Suggestions for additional study

1. Keep a notebook throughout the course. Cut out any articles on nutrition. Bring them to class for discussion and evaluation and then paste them in your notebook.
2. Make a list of your food intake for 3 days and analyze each day in accordance with The Basic Four Food Groups.
3. At some time during the first half of the course, each student gives a special report on some phase of nutrition. Students may choose a subject from the phase of nutrition that interests them most. This report is given before the class and then placed in the notebook.

References

Food and Nutrition Board, National Academy of Sciences–National Research Council: Recommended dietary allowances, ed. 8, Washington, D. C., 1974, The Academy.

Guthrie, H. A.: Introductory nutrition, ed. 4, St. Lous, 1979, The C. V. Mosby Co., Chapters 1, 14.

Robinson, C. H.: Basic nutrition and diet therapy, ed. 3, New York, 1975, The Macmillan Co.

Williams, S. R.: Nutrition and diet therapy, ed. 3, St. Louis, 1977, The C. V. Mosby Co., Chapters 11, 15.

Williams, S. R.: Essentials of nutrition and diet therapy, ed. 2 St. Louis, 1978, The C. V. Mosby Co., Chapters 1, 9.

2

Carbohydrates

The main function of carbohydrate in nutrition is to provide energy. Under normal circumstances it supplies the primary fuel to meet about two thirds of an individual's total energy needs. When sufficient carbohydrate is not available in the food consumed, the body, after calling heavily on its stored glycogen, breaks down tissue fat and protein to meet its energy demands.

The ease with which carbohydrate is converted into glycogen greatly adds to its usefulness. Glycogen is found in several tissues of the body, but the main storehouses are the liver and muscles. Although the body's reserve of liver and muscle glycogen is not large, it is readily available for quick energy and is rapidly replaced.

Another important function of carbohydrate is its ability to spare protein metabolism. When the diet consists largely of carbohydrate, there is a much lower level of protein metabolism for energy than when the diet is composed of protein or fat alone, or both.

Carbohydrate foods include starches such as grains and vegetables, and fruits and other sweets. These foods provide our chief source of energy. They form from 50% to 60% of the American diet and are the cheapest form of fuel for producing energy in the body. Milk also contains carbohydrate as milk sugar (lactose) but is generally classified with protein foods since milk protein is of high biological value.

The United States is one of the big consumers of sugar and products made from sugar. Sweets in general are an expensive and nutritionally poor source of calories. Too much sugar in the diet dulls the appetite for foods that are needed to supply the necessary vitamins and minerals, is irritating to the inner lining of the stomach, and ferments readily, causing gas. When sugars are absorbed in amounts that exceed the body's ability to use the accumulated glycogen, they are converted into fat and stored as such.

The carbohydrates are divided into three groups: monosaccharides, disaccharides, and polysaccharides.

The two most common *monosaccharides*, or single sugars, are glucose, which is derived mainly from the digestion of starch, and fructose, which is found abundantly in fruits. The amount of sugar in fruits depends somewhat on the degree of ripeness. As the fruit ripens, some of the starch changes to sugar. The single sugars require no digestion. They are quickly absorbed from the intestine into the bloodstream and are carried to the liver, where they are converted by liver enzymes into glycogen, a form of carbohydrate similar in structure to starch (thus sometimes called "animal starch"), or used for immediate energy needs.

The most common of the *disaccharides*, or double sugars, are sucrose and lactose. Sucrose is found in common sugar—granulated, powdered, or brown. Molasses, a by-product of sugar manufacturing, is also a form of sucrose. Lactose is the sugar present in milk and is the only common sugar not found in plants. It is less soluble and less sweet than sucrose. It remains in the intestines longer than other sugars and encourages the growth of certain useful bacteria. Lactose forms approximately 40% of milk solids. It is formed in the mammary glands. There is 4.8% lactose in cow's milk and 7% in human milk. Studies have shown that lactose favors calcium and phosphorus assimilation. Lactose is often added to fruit juices to increase their caloric value. It is possible to add more lactose than any other sugar to a beverage because it is not as sweet as the others and does not detract from the palatability of the product.

Polysaccharides are composed of many molecules of simple sugars and include starches, glycogen, cellulose, and hemicellulose.

Starches are found in grains and vegetables and in minute amounts in fruits. Starches are more complex than sugars and require a longer time to digest. In order for starch to be promptly used by the body, the outer membrane must be broken down by grinding or cooking. Heat, especially if moisture is present, causes the outer membrane to break apart, and the starch granules will then absorb the water and swell. Long application of dry heat will also cause starch to break down.

Glycogen, or "animal starch," is found in the liver and muscles. The glycogen of the liver is broken down to glucose, which is released into a bloodstream when needed for energy in the body.

Cellulose, a source of dietary fiber, is another important form of carbohydrate in our food. It is the fiber that forms the framework of our fruits, vegetables, and cereals. We lack the necessary enzymes to digest it, so it has no direct nutrient value as do other carbohydrates, but its indigestibility is its most important asset. It furnishes the bulk essential for the normal peristaltic action necessary for elimination of waste products. A normal person requires approximately 6 grams of cellulose a day. If a person eats two vegetables, two fruits, and four servings of whole-grain bread or cereal, as listed in The Basic Four Food Groups, he will have eaten 6 grams of cellulose.

Hemicellulose, another form of fiber, is closely related to cellulose but is somewhat different in chemical structure. The most common types are agar, alginate, and pectin. Agar, obtained from seaweed, has the ability to absorb many times its weight in water. It is often used in the treatment of constipation. Alginate, also obtained from seaweed, is used in making commercial ice cream to give it a smooth texture. Pectins, obtained from fruits, are useful for their jelling properties. Pectin is also used in the treatment of diarrhea because its absorbs the toxins and bacteria in the intestines and also adds bulk to the contents of the intestines.

We need sufficient carbohydrate in our diet to supply us with heat and energy so that our protein will not have to be diverted to energy needs. Heat and energy requirements will be supplied first; therefore, it is necessary to have enough carbohydrate in the diet to take care of these needs adequately, sparing the protein for its primary use—that of building and maintaining tissues. It is important that the carbohydrate be consumed at the same time as the protein, or the sparing action of the carbohydrate is lessened.

The body keeps a reasonably constant level of glucose in the blood. The glucose is used as a source of energy wherever it is needed. It is carried to the muscles, where it is used to restore the glycogen that is broken down to supply energy for muscular use, and to the nervous system. Almost one third of the carbohydrate in a healthy individual is in the liver, stored as glycogen to serve as a ready source of glucose for other parts of the body.

Some carbohydrate is also necessary for the normal metabolism of other nutrients. When, in the absence of sufficient carbohydrate, the body is forced to burn too much fat, a condition known as acidosis appears. The products of incomplete fat oxidation in the cells are strong acids (ketones) that upset the normal acid-base balance of the body.

Questions on carbohydrates

1. What are the chief sources of carbohydrates?
2. What are the chief functions of carbohydrates?
3. Why is it not good to have too much sugar in the diet?
4. What are the three principal groups of carbohydrates?
5. Where are the single sugars found?
6. What is sucrose?
7. Which sugar is not found in plants?
8. How does lactose differ from other carbohydrates?
9. What is necessary to make starch more readily available to the body?
10. What is glycogen and where is it found?
11. What is cellulose and why is it advantageous in the normal diet?
12. How may a person be assured of receiving enough cellulose in his diet?
13. Where is cellulose found?
14. What use is made of agar, alginate, and pectin?
15. Why do we need an adequate amount of carbohydrate in the diet?

Suggestions for additional study

1. Cut pictures from magazines illustrating carbohydrate foods and put in notebook.
2. Add 2 tbs. lactose to 1/2 cup orange juice and compare the taste with that of plain orange juice.

3. Compare the taste of a ripe banana with that of one only partially ripe and describe the difference.
4. Make a list of foods high in carbohydrates that are usually consumed between meals.
5. Read the labels on five different products in a grocery market and list the carbohydrate value of each.

References

Guthrie, H. A.: Introductory nutrition, ed. 4, St. Louis, 1979, The C. V. Mosby Co.

Williams, S. R.: Nutrition and diet therapy, ed. 3, St. Louis, 1977, The C. V. Mosby Co., Chapter 2.

Williams, S. R.: Essentials of nutrition and diet therapy, ed. 2, St. Louis, 1978, The C. V. Mosby Co., Chapter 2.

3

Proteins

Protein is the fundamental structural material of every cell in the body. In fact, the largest percentage of the body (with the exception of water) is made up of protein that must be constantly repaired and replaced. Protein not only makes up the bulk of the muscles, internal organs, brain, nerves, skin, hair, and nails but also is a part of the hormones and enzymes that are so important to the functioning of the body. Protein is a normal constituent of all body fluids except bile and urine. If needed, proteins may furnish heat and energy to the body. The main function of proteins, however, is to repair worn-out or wasted tissue and build new tissue. They also combine with iron to form the hemoglobin in the blood. Hemoglobin, a protein compound, gives the red coloring to the corpuscles. About 10,000 atoms make up a hemoglobin molecule; about 100 million molecules make up a corpuscle.

Because our only source of protein is food, it is important that we receive the proper kind and amount of proteins in our daily diet.

Protein is an essential element in the performance of the following additional functions:

1. Regulating osmotic pressures within body fluids to maintain normal circulation and water balance
2. Manufacturing hormones and enzymes
3. Building antibodies with which the body fights infection

Unlike carbohydrates and fats, which contain no nitrogen, proteins contain approximately 16% nitrogen, and some proteins contain small but valuable amounts of sulfur, phosphorus, iron, and iodine. The amount of protein consumed and ulitized by the body is measured by the amount of nitrogen consumed in the protein and the amount excreted in the urine. One gram of urinary nitrogen results from the digestion of 6.25 grams of protein. Therefore, if for every 6.25 grams of protein consumed, 1 gram of nitrogen is excreted in the urine, the body is said to be in nitrogen balance, which is the normal pattern.

A positive nitrogen balance means that the body has excreted less nitrogen than it has taken in and is therefore retaining nitrogen. This situation may occur during rapid growth in infancy, childhood, or adolescence, or during pregnancy or lactation, or it may occur in persons who have been malnourished and are subsequently being "built back up" with increased nourishment. In such cases protein is being retained within the body to supply its increased needs.

A negative nitrogen balance means that the body has excreted more nitrogen than it has consumed, indicating that the body is breaking down some of the body protein. Failure to keep the body in nitrogen balance may not become apparent for some time, but it will eventually cause loss of muscle tissue, impairment of body organs and body functions, and increased susceptibility to infection. In children, growth is retarded.

Proteins are made up of small building units or compounds known as amino acids, which are joined in various specific combinations to form specific proteins. In the digestive tract protein is broken down into amino acids, which are reassembled within the body in the proper order to form the needed body protein. There are twenty-two known amino acids at present, eight of which are essential in the diet because the body cannot synthesize them.

An adult diet must provide the following eight essential amino acids: tryptophan, threonine, isoleucine, leucine, lysine, methionine, phenylalanine, and valine. Children seem to also need histidine for normal growth. Arginine is synthesized in the body but not in an amount sufficient to meet the demands of normal growth.

Proteins are divided into two groups: complete proteins and incomplete proteins.

The complete proteins contain all of the eight essential amino acids, which the body cannot synthesize, in sufficient quantities for normal growth and maintenance. Complete proteins are sometimes spoken of as proteins of high biological value, which means that they supply all the amino acids needed for building body tissues. In general, all proteins from animal sources, such as meats, poultry, fish, eggs, milk, and cheese, provide high-quality protein in liberal amounts. Gelatin, although an animal product, is not a complete protein.

Incomplete proteins are those that contain many amino acids but not all the essential ones in sufficient amounts. However, they are a very important supplement to the complete proteins. These proteins are found in cereals, legumes, and certain nuts and seeds. By including these proteins in the diet, one can decrease the amount of animal proteins needed.

Fortunately, most of our foods contain a mixture of proteins that supplement each other. We combine several foods in one meal, and the protein in one supplements the protein in the others. Bread and milk, cereal and milk, and meat, cheese, or egg sandwiches are very logical as well as very useful combinations.

The amino acids that are incomplete in vegetable protein are present in adequate amounts in meat, milk, and eggs, and it has been found that the overall protein value is improved when foods of animal origin are eaten along with foods of vegetable origin.

In general, the proteins in one food will supplement those contained in another food more efficiently if they are eaten at the same time. For instance, the proteins of bread and those of milk supplement each other better if taken at the same time. One of the important facts of protein nutrition is that although there is no storage of amino acids in the body as such, a metabolic "pool" of amino acids is maintained in the liver to meet constant cell needs. This general metabolic resource helps to assure a provision for synthesis of needed tissue proteins.

The body makes such combinations of the amino acids as are needed at the time. Each body cell has its own specific composition; therefore, it can use only its own particular type and amount of amino acid. The time element is important in protein metabolism. It is necessary that all the required amino acids be presented to a particular tissue by the bloodstream at the same time. It is not possible for one of the needed amino acids to be presented several hours later and find the other essential amino acid waiting to help do the job. Therefore, it becomes important that some form of complete animal protein, or complementary combinations of incomplete plant proteins, be included in each meal to ensure that the necessary amino acids for repairing the cells are will present in the bloodstream when needed.

Current research indicates that the so-called specific dynamic action of protein is far more insignificant than was formerly assumed. In other words, a high-protein diet does not make the body "burn up" more calories than a normal diet does.

Food should contain sufficient protein to provide an intake well above actual needs to ensure an adequate supply of the essential amino acids contained in the complete proteins. The necessary margin of safety means that usually there will be some surplus. After all the protein needs of the body have been met, the amino acids not needed are carried back to the liver, where they are divided into two substances. Approximately one half is converted into urea in the liver and excreted through the kidneys, and the other half is routed through the same channels as carbohydrates and is used to provide energy for body needs.

Many metabolic functions of amino acids are now recognized. For instance, methionine serves as a source of "labile methyl groups" for the synthesis of choline or creatine. Arginine is likewise involved in the synthesis of creatine. Phenylalanine furnishes the nucleus for the synthesis of thyroxine. It is evident, then, that there are additions to the more general functions of amino acids that were recognized in classical metabolic physiology.

The protein requirements may be modified by certain pathological conditions or circumstances. For example, the protein level should be high before surgery to prevent liver damage due to the toxic effects of the anesthetic and to

Table 3-1. Required amounts of protein per day*

Men (154 lb.)	51	grams
Women (128 lb.)	46	grams
Women (pregnant, last 4½ mo.)	76	grams
Women (lactating)	66	grams
Infants		
0 to 6 mo.		2.2 grams per kilogram of body weight
6 to 12 mo.		2.0 grams per kilogram of body weight
Children		
1 to 3 yr.	23	grams
4 to 6 yr.	30	grams
7 to 10 yr.	36	grams
Boys		
11 to 14 yr.	45	grams
15 to 18 yr.	54	grams
Girls		
11 to 14 yr.	44	grams
15 to 18 yr.	48	grams

*From Food and Nutrition Board, National Academy of Sciences—National Research Council: Recommended dietary allowances, ed. 8, Washington, D.C., 1974, The Academy, p. 103.

Table 3-2. Foods high in protein

Food	Approximate amount	Protein (gm.)
Beef, chuck roast	3 oz. cooked	23.4
Beef, hamburger	3 oz. cooked	20.5
Beef, round	3 oz. cooked	24.7
Beef, club steak	4 oz. cooked	27.6
Lamb leg	3 oz. cooked	21.6
Liver (beef, calf, and pork)	3 oz. cooked	20.4
Pork loin	3 oz. cooked	20.7
Ham	3 oz. cooked	20.7
Veal, leg or shoulder	3 oz. cooked	25.2
Chicken	¼ broiler	22.4
Chicken, fryer	½ breast (4 oz. raw)	26.9
Chicken, hen, stewed	1 thigh or ½ breast	26.5
Duck, roasted	3 slices (3½ × 2¾ × ¼)	20.6
Goose, roasted	3 slices (3½ × 2¾ × ¼)	25.3
Turkey	3 slices (3½ × 2¼ × ¼)	27.8
Haddock	3 oz. cooked	20.2
Halibut	3 oz. cooked	21.0
Oysters	6 medium	15.1
Salmon	⅔ cup	20.5
Scallops	5 to 6 medium	23.8
Tuna	½ cup	15.9
Peanut butter	4 tbs.	15.9
Milk	1 cup	8.5
Cottage cheese	5 to 6 tbs.	19.5
American cheddar cheese	1 oz.	7.1

provide necessary resources for healing. Extra amounts of protein are also needed after surgery and for patients with burns or other conditions necessitating the building of new tissue. Although strenuous physical labor does not actually increase the need for added protein, an increased amount of protein, along with an increased amount of calories from other sources, is more satisfying.

Protein as protein is not stored in the body, but in severe protein deficiency, the body cells will release a part of their tissue protein, which makes it important to have an optimum amount of protein in the diet at all times.

The amounts of daily protein recommended by the Food and Nutrition Board are given in Table 3-1. These amounts are designed for the maintenance of good nutrition in a healthy person who is engaged in moderate physical activity.

Of this protein intake, the percentage of complete proteins should be 33% for adults and 50% to 60% for children. Because they are growing, the protein needs of boys and girls up to the age of 20 years are greater per pound of body weight than those of an adult. The protein requirements of boys and girls have little variation for the first 12 years. When they reach adolescence, the protein intake should be somewhat higher for boys than for girls, as shown in Table 3-1. A variety of foods high in protein is shown in Table 3-2. These foods may be used in many ways in planning menus.

A high-protein diet should contain approximately 100 grams of protein in a day's menu, which, translated into foods, for example, would mean three glasses of milk, two large servings of meat, fish, or poultry, and three eggs used either as such or in cooking, in addition to regular amounts of fruits, vegetables, and dessert.

A low-protein diet should contain no more than 40 grams of protein in a day's diet, which would mean the person could have, in addition to one serving of cereal, three slices of bread, green vegetables, fruits, and a choice of the following groups of protein foods:

1 cup milk	or	2 cups milk	or	1 cup milk and
1 egg and		and 1 egg		2 oz. meat
1 oz. meat				

Questions on proteins

1. Name the areas in the body that are made up largely of proteins.
2. What is the protein that gives the red color to blood?
3. What are the functions of protein in the body?
4. Name the eight essential amino acids.
5. What minerals are found in the different proteins?
6. Define nitrogen balance, positive nitrogen balance, and negative nitrogen balance.
7. How many essential amino acids have been discovered to date?
8. What is a complete protein, and where are the complete proteins found?
9. What is meant by high biological value?

10. What are incomplete proteins, and where are they found?
11. Why is the time element important in protein metabolism?
12. Why is it advisable to provide a protein intake above actual needs?
13. What happens to excess protein?
14. When is it advisable to give a high-protein diet?
15. What percentage of the protein intake should be from complete proteins for adults, and what percentage for children? Why are the percentages different?
16. Which of the following foods would you use on a high-protein diet: cheese, peach, spinach, salmon, banana?
17. Underline the complete proteins in the following list: Cream of Wheat, eggs, applesauce, roast beef, coffee, milk.
18. List your protein intake for 1 day, indicating which are complete and which are incomplete.

Suggestions for additional study

1. Place pictures cut from magazines illustrating complete proteins on one page of your notebook and those showing incomplete proteins on another page.
2. List the foods rich in protein that you would normally consume at each of the three daily meals.
3. Prepare for the class a display of actual foods, showing those containing complete proteins and those containing incomplete proteins. Use these foods to demonstrate how you would plan a vegetarian diet to assure adequate complete protein.
4. Plan a high-protein diet and a low-protein diet for 3 days.

References

Church, C. F., and Church, H. N.: Food values of portions commonly used, ed. 11, Philadelphia, 1970, J. B. Lippincott Co.

Food and Nutrition Board, National Academy of Sciences–National Research Council: Recommended dietary allowances, ed. 8, Washington, D.C., 1974, The Academy.

Guthrie, H. A.: Introductory nutrition, ed. 4, St. Louis, 1979, The C. V. Mosby Co.

Williams, S. R.: Nutrition and diet therapy, ed. 3, St. Louis, 1977, The C. V. Mosby Co., Chapter 4.

Williams, S. R.: Essentials of nutrition and diet therapy, ed. 2, St. Louis, 1978, The C. V. Mosby Co., Chapter 5.

4

Fats

Fats are composed of oils that are liquid at room temperature and of fats that are solid and semisolid.

Not all fats are visible. Therefore, for practical purposes we classify them as visible and invisible fats. The visible fats include lard, butter, margarine, shortenings, salad oils, and the visible fat of meat. The invisible fats include those in milk, cheese, eggs, nuts, and meat. Even when all of the visible fat has been removed from meat, an average of 6% of fat surrounding the muscle fibers will remain.

Margarine and shortenings are made from relatively less expensive vegetable oils, such as cottonseed oil, soybean oil, and corn oil, by the introduction of hydrogen into the fat molecule under carefully controlled conditions. Margarine is then further processed by being churned with cultured milk to give the flavor of butter. It is usually fortified the vitamins A and D. Nutritionally, fortified margarine is the equivalent of butter and has the same caloric value as butter. Margarine, which is tasty as well as economical, is 80% fat and is fortified with vitamin A to supply a minimum of 15,000 units per pound (U.S.P.).

The average American eats approximately 100 pounds of fat a year, which provides about 40% of his total calories. This amount of fat is in excess of that needed by the average person. Not more than 20% to 30% of an average diet need be in the form of fats. If 20% of the total calories come from fat, an adequate amount of the essential fatty acids to meet the physiological needs of the body will be present. On a 2,000-calorie diet, a person would still be getting 45 to 50 grams of fat. It has been demonstrated in Asia and eastern Europe that even 20% to 25% fat in the diet is not necessary to the health of all persons.

Fats serve several purposes in the diet. Some act as carriers of the fat-soluble vitamins, A, D, E, and K, and favor absorption of fat-soluble factors. They all give a feeling of satisfaction to the meal, due partly to the slow rate of digestion of fats and partly to the flavor they give to foods.

The fat not needed for immediate use is stored as fatty tissue to be used in an emergency. This storage of fat is beneficial for several reasons: It assists in regulating body temperature because the layer of fat beneath the skin acts as a nonconductor and prevents excessive radiation or loss of body heat. It protects the body from mechanical injury and acts as a support to the vital organs.

A particular fatty acid, linoleic acid, is recognized as the main essential fatty acid because the body cannot synthesize it and it is vital to body processes. Two other fatty acids, linolenic acid and arachidonic acid, have been called essential fatty acids but are not actually dietary essentials, because the body can synthesize them. The essential one, linoleic acid, is found primarily in vegetable oils.

The digestibility of fats varies somewhat. Butter digests more completely than meat fats. Fried foods, especially those that are saturated with fat, digest more slowly than boiled or baked foods. Fried food cooked at too high a temperature is more difficult to digest; substances in that fat break down into irritating substances. Fried foods should be used sparingly, and the temperature of the fat used in frying should be carefully controlled.

Fats are a more concentrated source of energy than carbohydrates, yielding two and one-fourth times as many calories per unit of weight. However, fats are still a more expensive source of calories than carbohydrate foods.

Cholesterol is a complex fat-related compound found in practically all body tissues, especially in the brain and nerve tissues, the bile, the blood, and the liver, where most of the cholesterol is synthesized. Cholesterol is synthesized within the body mainly in the intestinal walls and the liver according to need, metabolic balances, and dietary intake. It has been estimated that the human body normally synthesizes about 2 grams of cholesterol daily.

At present much research is being done on the relationship of dietary cholesterol to atherosclerosis and coronary disease, and on the reasons why cholesterol from large molecules that contain cholesterol and fats (triglycerides) with plasma protein, compounds called *lipoproteins*, is deposited on the walls of the blood vessels. Various studies seem to indicate that a high consumption of dietary cholesterol and animal fats may lead to abnormal levels of cholesterol bodies in the blood in susceptible individuals and that an increased intake of plant fats, especially those containing linoleic acid, lowers the blood cholesterol level.

A high blood cholesterol level does not necessarily mean that large cholesterol bodies are deposited on the walls of the blood vessels and vice versa. However, a blood cholesterol level that is higher than 240 mg. per 100 ml. should be a warning sign that trouble may possibly be just around the corner. It would be wise to have a count taken every few months.

Many physicians and nutritionists are prescribing a low-cholesterol, low-fat diet. At least it is a step forward, for the American people ordinarily consume a very high percentage of fat in the diet. As was stated, approximately 40% of the calories consumed are derived from fat. The countries that have a lower fat intake show a much lower incidence of coronary disease. The American public would do well to cut its fat intake from 40% to 20% or 30% and thereby reduce the caloric intake and perhaps lower the blood cholesterol level. There is less atherosclerosis in countries where the use of saturated (animal) fats is low and unsaturated (plant) fats are used. This is the case in Japan. Surveys made in Italy, Spain, Africa, and other countries where the people's intake of fat is approximately 20% show that there are lower cholesterol levels and less atherosclerosis.

One point on which all physicians and nutritionists agree is that being over-weight tends to increase the cholesterol content of the blood and the risk of heart disease. Therefore, a middle-aged or older person who is overweight and who also has a high blood cholesterol level will find it advisable to reduce both his weight and his consumption of fats, especially animal fats. The cholesterol content of some foods is given in Table 4-1.

The foods that are lowest in cholesterol are fruits, vegetables, bread, cereals, skim milk, buttermilk, cottage cheese, jelly, syrup, and sugar.

Low-cholesterol, low-fat diet (1,600 calories)

Include these foods daily:
  2 cups skim milk
  6 oz. lean meat, fish, shellfish except shrimp, or poultry
  1/2 cup cereal, whole grain or enriched
  6 slices bread, whole grain or enriched
  3 tsp. margarine, made from vegetable oil
  1 serving potatoes
  3 servings vegetables, one raw
  3 servings fruit, one citrus
Foods to avoid:
  Egg yolks
  Whole milk
  Butter
  Cheese made from whole milk
  Cream
  Organ meats of any kind
  Shrimp
  Ice cream made with whole milk
  Pies made with lard
Foods that may be used:
  Lean meats, 4 to 6 oz. a day
  Skim milk
  Vegetables
  Fruit
  Breads and cereals, especially whole grains
  Margarine, 3 pats a day
  Egg white

The three kinds of fats important to the cholesterol level are (1) *saturated*

Table 4-1. Cholesterol content of foods*

Food item	Size of serving	Cholesterol per serving (mg.)
Muscle meats		
Beef, round		
Medium fat	3⅓ oz.	125
Lean	3⅓ oz.	95
Lamb	3⅓ oz.	70
Veal	3⅓ oz.	65 to 140
Organ meats		
Liver		
Beef	3⅓ oz.	320
Calf	3⅓ oz.	360
Lamb	3⅓ oz.	610
Pork	3⅓ oz.	420
Sweetbreads	3⅓ oz.	280
Fish		
Shellfish		
Crab	3⅓ oz.	145
Oysters	3⅓ oz.	230 to 470
Shrimp	3⅓ oz.	150
Cod	3⅓ oz.	50
Salmon	3⅓ oz.	60
Sardines	1¾ oz.	35
Poultry		
Chicken, light	3⅓ oz.	90
Chicken, dark	3⅓ oz.	60
Duck	3⅓ oz.	70
Turkey	3⅓ oz.	75
Cheese		
American	2 oz.	96
American, processed	2 oz.	93
Swiss, processed	2 oz.	87
Velveeta	2 oz.	96
Miscellaneous		
Butter	1 tbs.	40
Egg yolk, fresh	1	333
Milk, whole	1 cup	26
Milk, skim	1 cup	1

*Data compiled from Okey, R.: Cholesterol content of food, J. Am. Diet. Assoc. **21:**341, 1945; Church, C. F., and Church, H. N.: Food values of portions commonly used, ed. 11, Philadelphia, 1970, College Offset Press.

fats, found in butter, whole milk, bacon, and fatty meats, which promote the body's production of cholesterol; (2) *monounsaturated fats,* mostly oleic acid, which forms the basic fat in olive oil and has no apparent effect on the blood cholesterol level; and (3) *polyunsaturated fats,* found in most vegetable oils and some fish (salmon, mackerel, and herring). An important component of polyunsaturated fats is linoleic acid, which lowers the blood cholesterol level, apparently by playing some key role in the transport and metabolism of cholesterol. The precise nature of this relationship is as yet not clearly understood.

In most people with high plasma cholesterol levels, a diet that contains an adequate amount of polyunsaturated fats, with a sufficient reduction of saturated fat and dietary cholesterol, will usually reduce the cholesterol level.

The cause of atherosclerosis is not clear. It is likely that fats are but one among several important causes. Until the evidence is more complete, persons with atherosclerosis should avoid an excess of cholesterol and animal fats.

Questions on fats

1. Name three visible fats.
2. Name three sources of invisible fats.
3. How is margarine made? How does it compare nutritionally with butter?
4. What percentage of the total calories in the average diet should be in the form of fat?
5. What purposes do fats serve in the diet?
6. What is the main essential fatty acid? Where is it found?
7. Compare the digestibility of butter or margarine with meat fats.
8. What precautions should be taken in frying foods and why?
9. Where is cholesterol found in the body?
10. List six foods high in cholesterol and six foods low in cholesterol.

Suggestions for additional study

1. Place pictures of foods containing visible fats on one page of your notebook and pictures of foods containing invisible fats on another page.
2. An average person will consume approximately 90 grams of fat, whereas a person on a low-to-moderate fat intake will use approximately 45 grams. Illustrate this point by placing 6 tbs. (90 grams) of a concentrated fat in one jar and 3 tbs. (45 grams) in another. Discuss the difference from a health and a caloric standpoint (90 grams of fat will contain 810 calories, whereas 45 grams will contain only 405 calories).
3. Plan a low-cholesterol, low-fat diet.

References

Guthrie, H. A.: Introductory nutrition, ed. 4, St. Louis, 1979, The C. V. Mosby Co.

Williams, S. R.: Nutrition and diet therapy, ed. 3, St. Louis, 1977, The C. V. Mosby Co.

Williams, S. R.: Essentials of nutrition and diet therapy, ed. 2, St. Louis, 1978, The C. V. Mosby Co.

5

Energy requirements

Energy is needed whenever any work is performed by the body. The actions can be voluntary or involuntary. Voluntary action refers to such activities as walking or any other movements that are consciously performed. Involuntary action consists of those activities that go on within the body and are not consciously performed, such as circulation, respiration, digestion, and absorption.

Both kinds of action require an expenditure of energy that must come from food. Therefore, the body must be supplied with fuel in the form of food in sufficient amounts to give energy for work and to keep the body warm. If sufficient food to supply the energy requirements and to furnish heat for the body is not consumed, the body will then borrow from its reserve fat. The average daily food intake should equal the daily energy requirements, except in obesity, in which the intake should be less than the daily energy needs in order to burn up the surplus fatty tissue.

The calorie is a measure of the energy that is produced by the burning, or oxidation, of food. (In the metric system the unit of measure for energy is called the joule.) In common usage the fuel values of the energy-producing foods are as follows:

Carbohydrates	4 calories per gram
Proteins	4 calories per gram
Fats	9 calories per gram

Humans spend the energy from their food in the necessary activity of the various organs of the body, in mechanical work, in the regulation of body temperature, and in the process of growth and repair of the body. The total chemical changes that occur during these activities are called metabolism. This exchange of energy is usually expressed in calories.

A basal metabolism test is taken when a person is at complete rest, although awake, in a room where the temperature is comfortable, 12 hours after any food has been consumed and several hours after strenuous exercise. The normal rate of basal metabolism varies somewhat according to the size and shape of the body, the age of the person, and the degree of activity of the thyroid gland. If

Table 5-1. Calories needed for average woman in different activities

Form of activity	Calories per hour, including basal needs
Sleeping	56
Sitting quietly	85
Standing relaxed	90
Standing at attention	96
Light exercise	143
Active exercise	244
Walking moderately fast	254
Walking downstairs	307
Walking upstairs	935

there is more than a 10% variance from the normal basal rate, an effort should be made to determine the cause.

The average basal energy requirement for a man is 1,650 calories daily and for a woman, 1,350 calories.

For the voluntary work of the body, the number of calories required depends largely on the degree of physical activity. The body weight of the person is also a determining factor. Mental work does not increase caloric needs. The varying amounts of calories needed for different activities for an average woman weighing 130 pounds are shown in Table 5-1.

Every movement, even a slight one, calls for calories to be used. Two individuals may do the same job, yet one will burn more calories than the other because of wasted motions.

An estimate of the energy needs of a moderately active woman may be made by allowing 18 calories per pound of ideal weight and of a moderately active man by allowing 20.5 calories for each pound of ideal weight. For the man who is doing strenuous labor, the allowance may need to be raised to as high as 28 calories for each pound of ideal weight. Example:

$$\begin{array}{r} \text{Ideal weight of woman} = 120 \text{ pounds} \\ \times \quad 18 \\ \hline 2,160 \text{ calories} \end{array}$$

Thus, 2,160 calories are needed by a woman weighing 120 pounds in order to maintain her present weight if she is moderately active. If by necessity or choice she becomes less active, she will need to lower her caloric intake accordingly.

Energy needs can be estimated only approximately because of the varying amounts of activity and time spent in activity and in resting.

A person's ideal weight at 25 years of age should be maintained throughout his life. The caloric intake should be gradually reduced from 30 years of age onward in order to maintain this ideal weight. Calories should be reduced by ap-

Table 5-2. Approximate caloric allowances for ages 1 month to 19 years

Age	Calories per pound	Age	Calories per pound	Age	Calories per pound
Infants		Children		Boys	
1 to 3 mo.	54.5	1 to 3 yr.	45.0	13 to 15 yr.	30.0
4 to 9 mo.	49.5	4 to 6 yr.	40.0	16 to 19 yr.	25.5
10 to 12 mo.	45.5	7 to 9 yr.	40.0	Girls	
		10 to 12 yr.	32.0	13 to 15 yr.	24.3
				16 to 19 yr.	20.0

Table 5-3. Mean heights and weights and recommended energy intake*

Category	Age (years)	Weight		Height		Energy needs (with range)	
		kg	lb	cm	in	kcal	MJ
Infants	0.0-0.5	6	13	60	24	kg × 115 (95-145)	kg × .48
	0.5-1.0	9	20	71	28	kg × 105 (80-135)	kg × .44
Children	1-3	13	29	90	35	1300 (900-1800)	5.5
	4-6	20	44	112	44	1700 (1300-2300)	7.1
	7-10	28	62	132	52	2400 (1650-3300)	10.1
Males	11-14	45	99	157	62	2700 (2000-3700)	11.3
	15-18	66	145	176	69	2800 (2100-3900)	11.8
	19-22	70	154	177	70	2900 (2500-3300)	12.2
	23-50	70	154	178	70	2700 (2300-3100)	11.3
	51-75	70	154	178	70	2400 (2000-2800)	10.1
	76+	70	154	178	70	2050 (1650-2450)	8.6
Females	11-14	46	101	157	62	2200 (1500-3000)	9.2
	15-18	55	120	163	64	2100 (1200-3000)	8.8
	19-22	55	120	163	64	2100 (1700-2500)	8.8
	23-50	55	120	163	64	2000 (1600-2400)	8.4
	51-75	55	120	163	64	1800 (1400-2200)	7.6
	76+	55	120	163	64	1600 (1200-2000)	6.7
Pregnancy						+ 300	
Lactation						+ 500	

The data in this table have been assembled from the observed median heights and weights of children shown in [Table 1-2], together with desirable weights for adults given in [Table B] for the mean heights of men (70 inches) and women (64 inches) between the ages of 18 and 34 years as surveyed in the U.S. population (HEW/NCHS data).

The energy allowances for the young adults are for men and women doing light work. The allowances for the two older age groups represent mean energy needs over these age spans, allowing for a 2% decrease in basal (resting) metabolic rate per decade and a reduction in activity of 200 kcal/day for men and women between 51 and 75 years, 500 kcal for mean over 75 years and 400 kcal for women over 75. The customary range of daily energy output is shown for adults in parentheses, and is based on a variation in energy needs of ± 400 kcal at any one age (see text and Garrow, 1978), emphasizing the wide range of energy intakes appropriate for any group of people.

Energy allowances for children through age 18 are based on median energy intakes of children these ages followed in longitudinal growth studies. The values in parentheses are 10th and 90th percentiles of energy intake, to indicate the range of energy consumption among children of these ages.

*From Recommended dietary allowances, revised 1979, Food and Nutrition Board, National Academy of Sciences–National Research Council, Washington, D.C.

proximately 3% from 30 to 40 years of age and by another 3% from 40 to 50 years of age. From 50 to 60 years of age, calories should be reduced by 7.5%, and from 60 to 70 years of age, by another 7.5%. From 70 to 80 years of age, calories should be reduced by 10%. If this measure is followed, a man who receives 3,200 calories at 25 years of age would receive 2,575 calories at 70 years of age.

Energy requirements for children are greater per pound than for adults. The approximate caloric allowances per pound for the various age groups are given in Table 5-2. There should be a gradual addition of calories from one age group to another. A summary of the recommended daily calorie allowances, as listed in the 1979 revisions of the National Research Council, is shown in Table 5-3.

Questions on energy requirements

1. What is the difference between voluntary and involuntary actions of the body?
2. When is it advisable to have the daily food intake less than the daily energy requirements?
3. How many calories does 1 gram of carbohydrate produce? One gram of protein? One gram of fat?
4. Under what conditions is the basal metabolism test made?
5. What is meant by the basal metabolism rate?
6. What are some of the causes of normal variations in the basal rate in different persons?
7. What is the basal metabolism rate of the average man? Of the average woman?
8. Does mental work increase caloric needs?
9. Determine the number of calories needed by a woman whose ideal weight is 130 pounds.
10. Calculate the number of calories needed by a 175-pound man at hard labor.

Suggestions for additional study

1. Figure the number of calories you would need to maintain your own ideal weight.
2. If the composition of one slice of bread is 2 grams of protein, 1 gram of fat, and 12 grams of carbohydrate, what is the caloric value of that slice of bread?
3. Figure the caloric value of the following:

Food	Grams carbohydrates	Grams protein	Grams fat	Calories
1 cup milk	12	8	10	_____
¼ pint vanilla ice cream	15	3	9	_____
½ cup cooked carrots	7	2	0	_____
½ small grapefruit	10	0	0	_____

References

Food and Nutrition Board, National Academy of Sciences–National Research Council: Recommended dietary allowances, Washington, D.C., 1979, The Academy.

Guthrie, H. A.: Introductory nutrition, ed. 4, St. Louis, 1979, The C. V. Mosby Co.

Williams, S. R.: Nutrition and diet therapy, ed. 3, St. Louis, 1977, The C. V. Mosby Co.

Williams, S. R.: Essentials of nutrition and diet therapy, ed. 2, St. Louis, 1978, the C. V. Mosby Co.

6

Minerals

Minerals are found in relatively small amounts in the human body but are essential elements in the body structure and in the control of certain body functions. There are at least twenty known minerals in the body, all of which are important, although the function of some of the trace minerals is as yet unknown.

Four percent, by weight, of the body is mineral in some structural form, such as the bones and teeth, or as salts in the fluids of the body.

Minerals function in at least four ways within the body:

1. They are constituents of the bones and teeth, giving rigidity to their structure.

2. They play a part in maintaining the natural muscle and nerve reaction to a stimulus.

3. They help to maintain the acid-base balance and the fluid-electrolyte balance in the body.

4. They combine with organic compounds to make up certain hormones found in the body, such as iodine in thyroxine.

Although the various minerals are discussed separately, it must be remembered that their actions are interrelated in the body and that many times one mineral is combined with another to complete the reaction. For example, calcium and phosphorus function together to form calcium phosphate in the bones. The interrelation of minerals and vitamins is shown by the fact that, in addition to adequate calcium and phosphorus, we must have sufficient vitamin D for proper absorption and utilization of calcium.

The only minerals that require special attention in a normal person's diet are calcium, phosphorus, and iron. If a person eats a normal, well-balanced diet daily, he will usually receive the remaining minerals in adequate amounts.

However, in disease conditions, mineral constituents of the diet may need adjustment—for example, the additional iron needed in nutritional anemia.

Calcium is one of the minerals most likely to be deficient in the American diet. The body needs calcium throughout the life-span, especially during childhood, pregnancy, and lactation. If there is insufficient calcium in the diet, the blood will use the calcium in the bones to maintain the normal composition of the blood. This naturally causes the bones to become more fragile. A liberal amount of calcium taken throughout life will decrease the danger of fractures and broken bones in older age. Calcium metabolism moves slowly in an adult.

Calcium performs the following functions:

1. It builds bones and teeth (approximately 99% of the calcium is found in the bones). When calcium phosphate is removed from bone, the remaining bone tissue is as flexible as cartilage. When calcium phosphate is insufficient to produce a normal, healthy bone structure, bowed legs, enlarged ankles and wrists, and other deformities of the bone result.

2. It is essential to normal clotting of the blood.

3. It is essential to normal muscular contraction.

A decrease of calcium in the blood results in tetany, which is characterized by abnormal twitching of the muscles. If the blood calcium level becomes elevated, as in excess bone destruction, for example, the excess calcium is excreted in the urine.

Milk and milk products are the most important sources of readily available calcium. Some calcium is also present in most green leafy vegetables. There should be a margin of surplus in supplying the body with calcium and phosphorus since there is a certain amount of loss in cooking and in absorption.

The calcium in spinach, Swiss chard, and beet greens may not be available, because of the presence of oxalic acid, which interferes with calcium absorption. However, broccoli, kale, mustard greens, and turnip greens are high in calcium, and because they contain no oxalic acid, they are good sources of calcium.

The recommended daily allowance of calcium is 800 mg. per day for adults and 1,200 mg. for women during pregnancy and lactation. The recommended daily allowance for children is 800 to 1,200 mg. to provide especially for the rapid formation of bone. An adequate supply of vitamin D is also essential for the most efficient utilization of calcium and phosphorus. However, vitamin D can function only when adequate amounts of calcium and phosphorus are present. Milk enriched with vitamin D is the perfect source of all three of these important bone-producing materials.

All of the recommended amount of milk need not always be consumed as a beverage. It may be used in cooking puddings, soups, and sauces, or in milk products, such as ice cream and cheese. Valuable secondary sources of calcium include egg yolk, green leafy vegetables, legumes, nuts, and whole grains.

Phosphorus, aside from its function in forming calcium phosphate in the bone structure, is a constituent of every living cell.

Compounds of phosphorus are important in maintaining the acid-base balance of the body, in the metabolism of proteins, fats, and carbohydrates, in energy metabolism, and in the activity of vitamins and enzymes.

Phosphorus is so widely distributed in foods that it is much less likely to be deficient in the average diet.

Poultry, fish, meat, cereals, nuts, and legumes, as well as milk and milk products, contain phosphorus.

Iron is very important to the well-being of a person, although there is less than 5 grams in the body of a full-grown healthy person. Iron helps make up hemoglobin, the coloring matter of the red blood cells; it is the oxygen-bearing element in the blood, and it is an essential part of every cell in the body. Our bodies use iron very efficiently by conserving it and then reusing it again and again.

However, iron deficiencies can and do occur, such as in infancy when the reserve in the liver is gone and the dietary intake is not yet adequate. Iron deficiencies may also occur as a result of menstrual losses, pregnancy, or hemorrhage. Whenever red blood cells are lost by hemorrhage, the iron is also lost. In the National Research Council's 1968 revisions and continued in the 1979 revisions, the recommended allowances for iron were raised, especially for growth and for adolescent girls and women during their childbearing years. It is doubtful that a woman's ordinary diet can supply this larger quantity of iron, and fortification with iron supplements is probably desirable.

The recommended amount of iron for adults is 10 mg. per day for men and 18 mg. for all women during the childbearing years. Milk contains no iron. During the first 4 to 6 months of life, an infant has a sufficient supply of iron because a reserve of this mineral is stored in the liver of the infant during prenatal life. After this time the growing infant needs iron-rich solid food, such as enriched cereal and egg yolk, to avoid a "milk anemia." The recommended allowance for infants is 10 to 15 mg. Allowances for children are 15 mg. from 1 to 3 years of age, and 10 mg. from 3 to 10 years of age.

For girls, beginning at age 10 and continuing through their childbearing years, an allowance of 18 mg. is recommended. Girls are more likely than boys to be anemic at this time because of the menstruation process in girls. For boys 12 to 18 years of age, the period of rapid adolescent growth, 18 mg. of iron is recommended. Thereafter, during adulthood, 10 mg. daily is sufficient.

The richest sources of iron are liver and other organ meats, all muscle meats, egg yolks, green leafy vegetables, molasses, raisins, whole-grain bread, and whole-grain or enriched cereals. Molasses and raisins, while rich in iron, are seldom eaten in sufficient quantities to be of much value.

It has been found that the presence of copper is necessary in order for iron to be absorbed and used in the manufacture of hemoglobin. This further proves the interrelationships among the various minerals.

Iodine must be supplied continually if the thyroid gland is to function normally. Iodine is an essential nutrient for humans, and its major role in the human organism is the formation of the thyroid hormone. The amount of iodine in the body is approximately 25 mg., and most of it is in the thyroid gland.

About 100 to 200 mg. of iodine is needed daily in the diet to supply the basal metabolic requirement (about 25 μg.) that is absorbed. This need can be met by the regular use of iodized salt. Iodized salt contains 1 part of potassium iodide or sodium iodide for each 5,000 parts of salt. The iodide is stabilized in the salt in order to prevent loss.

The amount of iodine in vegetables depends on the amount of iodine in the soil in which they are grown. Vegetables grown in areas where the soil is low in iodine contain less iodine than those grown where there is more abundant iodine. In general, the most abundant supply of iodine in the soil is in those states bordering on the Atlantic coast and the Gulf of Mexico.

Ocean fish and shellfish are usually good sources of iodine.

Copper balance studies in humans reveal that a daily intake of 2 mg. of copper will maintain adults in balance. The human diet usually contains 2 to 4 mg. of copper per day. It is difficult to prepare a diet that contains less than that amount of copper. The copper content of whole blood is about equally divided between the cells and the plasma. It ranges from 90 to 150 μg. per 100 ml. for men and 100 to 160 μg. per 100 ml. for women. Milk is very low in copper.

Fluorine plays some role in dental health. In population groups having a small amount of fluorine in the water supply, the incidence of dental caries (tooth decay) is greatly reduced. Mottled enamel does not occur except when excessive quantities of fluoride are taken during the period of enamel formation. The fluorine content of the drinking water should not exceed 1 part per million.

In severe cases of fluoride intoxication from industrial exposures, there is calcification of ligaments and muscle attachments, gastrointestinal symptoms, and anemia. This condition has been reported from India, where drinking water has a fluoride content of 1 to 6 parts per million.

Questions on minerals

1. What purposes do minerals serve in the body?
2. What three minerals must we be certain to include in the diet in adequate amounts?
3. Why do we not have to watch the intake of other minerals so carefully?
4. What percentage of the weight of the body is mineral?
5. Where are the minerals found in the body?
6. What mineral is most likely to be deficient in the average American diet?
7. What is the most important source of calcium?
8. What are some sources of phosphorus?
9. How does the cooking process affect the amount of calcium and phosphorus in the food?
10. Where is most of the calcium and phosphorus found in the body?
11. What purpose does calcium serve in the blood?
12. What is the average daily requirement of calcium?
13. What food fulfills the requirements for calcium and phosphorus most completely and in the most readily available form?
14. What vitamin is concerned in the absorption and utilization of calcium and phosphorus?

15. Why is iron essential?
16. What foods are our best sources of iron?
17. What is the recommended amount of iron for adults?
18. What other mineral needs to be present in the liver for proper utilization of iron?
19. What is the average amount of iodine required by the body?
20. Where is iodine needed in the body?
21. What is the usual method of adding iodine to the diet?
22. Plan a day's menu that is rich in calcium and one that is rich in iron.
23. Of what importance is copper? Fluoride?

Suggestions for additional study

1. Put illustrations in your notebook of the foods that are richest in each of the minerals discussed in this chapter.
2. Prepare a chart showing the comparative values in calcium of several of the calcium-rich foods.
3. Using the food values listed in Table A (p. 174), compute the amount of iron in the following: (a) 3$^{1}/_3$ oz. beef liver, (b) 3 oz. round steak, (c) 1 tbs. molasses, (d) 1 tbs. raisins, (e) $^{1}/_2$ cup cooked kale, and (f) 6 stewed prunes.

References

Church, C. F.,and Church, H. N.: Food values of portions commonly used, ed. 11, Philadephia, 1970, J. B. Lippincott Co.

Food and Nutrition Board, National Academy of Sciences–National Research Council: Recommended dietary allowances, Washington, D.C., 1979, The Academy.

Guthrie, H. A.: Introductory nutrition, ed. 4, St. Louis, 1979, The C. V. Mosby Co.

Williams. S. R.: Nutrition and diet therapy, St. Louis, ed. 3, 1977, The C. V. Mosby Co.

Williams, S. R.: Essentials of nutrition and diet therapy, ed. 2, St. Louis, 1978, The C. V. Mosby Co.

7

Vitamins

Vitamins are organic compounds that regulate metabolism and make possible a more efficient utilization of carbohydrate, protein, and fat within the body. Vitamins themselves are totally lacking in caloric value. They are like the ignition spark, which furnishes no fuel but keeps the motor running in an orderly fashion. The total volume of vitamins that we require daily would barely fill a teaspoon, but they are essential to our existence.

Although all vitamins are essential, there are six vitamins to which we need pay special attention: vitamins A and D, ascorbic acid, thiamine, riboflavin, and niacin. The same foods that supply us with these six vitamins will also supply us with all the remaining vitamins. Each vitamin has a specific function to perform. Vitamins were first recognized by their absence rather than by their presence.

As early as 1753, Dr. James Lind, a surgeon in the British navy, discovered that scurvy, the curse of sailors, was caused by some dietary deficiency. On long voyages the sailors were obliged to live on very limited rations, with no fresh foods. It was learned that when certain fresh foods, such as lemons and limes, were given to the sailors, no one had scurvy. Thus originated the nickname of "limeys" for British sailors.

In 1906, Dr. Frederich Hopkins, working at Cambridge University in England, performed an experiment in which he fed a group of white rats a diet consisting of a synthetic mixture of proteins, fats, carbohydrates, mineral salts, and water, and the animals became sick and died. With the next group, Dr. Hopkins added milk to the purified ration, and the rats all lived and grew normally. Thus an important discovery was made—that there are accessory food factors present in *natural* foods that in some way are essential to life.

Much research on vitamins was necessary to make possible the knowledge from which we benefit today.

Vitamins will not relieve a physical illness that is not specifically caused by a lack of that particular vitamin. For instance, vitamin A would have no effect in relieving an abnormal condition in the eye unless the abnormal condition were caused by an insufficient amount of vitamin A.

The fat-soluble vitamins are vitamins A, D, K, and E.

The water-soluble ones are ascorbic acid (vitamin C) and the B-complex vitamins.

The word "deficiency" is usually used to indicate varying degrees of shortages—for example, mild, moderate, severe, or complete. Deficiency diseases are usually the result of deficiencies in more than one vitamin.

Subclinical deficiency states, which precede vitamin deficiency diseases, usually cause such vague symptoms that they are seldom brought to the attention of a physician. If these warning signs were heeded, more serious illness might often be averted.

Vitamins A and D, which are the only vitamins that the body is able to store in any quantity, are stored primarily in the liver. Some of the other vitamins are stored in such small amounts that it is important that a person be certain he has an adequate intake of each of the vitamins every day.

Several vitamins are needed for blood-building. Major blood "factories" in our bone marrow produce about 1 million new red blood cells every second to replace an equal number that have completed the life-span of approximately 4 months. Every budding red blood cell requires vitamin B_{12} and folic acid, another B vitamin, at vital stages of its growth.

FAT-SOLUBLE VITAMINS
Vitamin A

Functions. Vitamin A performs the following functions in the body:

1. It maintains the mucous membranes in the nose, throat, alimentary tract, eyes, and genitourinary tract in a healthy condition. A lack of vitamin A will aggravate an infection that may be present in the bronchial tubes, sinuses, or lungs.

2. It is essential in regenerating visual purple in the eye, a substance necessary for good vision. A mild deficiency in vitamin A will manifest itself by night blindness, slow adaptation to darkness, or glare blindness.

3. It is essential to growth. For example, lack of vitamin A, especially in growing children, retards skeletal growth.

4. It prevents xerosis, which is caused by a deficiency in vitamin A and is characterized by itching and burning of the eyes, with redness of the lids and some inflammation.

5. It prevents xerophthalmia, which is caused by a very severe deficiency in vitamin A and which often produces permanent blindness before the disease can be controlled.

Human requirements. The recommended daily allowance for the average adult is 800 μg. R.E. (retinol equivalents) for women and 1,000 μg. for men. The recommended daily allowance for a pregnant woman is 1,000 μg. R.E. during pregnancy and 1,200 μg. R.E. during lactation.

Recommended daily allowances for children are as follows:

Birth to 6 mo.	420 μg. R.E.	7 to 10 yr.	700 μg. R.E.
6 mo. to 1 yr.	400 μg. R.E.	11 to 22 yr.	
1 to 3 yr.	400 μg. R.E.	Males	1,000 μg. R.E.
4 to 6 yr.	500 μg. R.E.	Females	800 μg. R.E.

Sources. Among the best sources of preformed vitamin A (retinol) are fish liver oils, liver, egg yolk, butter, and cream. Carotene is a pigment in dark green and yellow vegetables and fruits that is changed into vitamin A within the body. Some good sources of carotene are carrots, leafy green vegetables, yellow corn, sweet potatoes, apricots, and peaches. Both carotene and preformed vitamin A require the presence of bile salts for proper absorption in the intestine. In the absence of bile, carotene and vitamin A are not absorbed from the intestinal tract unless bile salts are administered orally. The bile salts act as an antioxidant to protect and stabilize the easily oxidized vitamin, and they also provide a vehicle of transport through the intestinal wall.

Stability. Vitamin A is unstable in heat in contact with air. Cooking vegetables in an open kettle is more destructive to vitamin A than heating the product in a pan with a lid.

Heating for a shorter time at a higher temperature is less destructive to the vitamin than heating for a longer period at a lower temperature.

If fats are rancid or vegetables are wilted, the majority of vitamin A has been destroyed.

Vitamin D

Functions. The following body functions are performed by vitamin D:

1. It is essential in the proper absorption and metabolism of calcium and phosphorus to produce normal growth of bone structures. However, vitamin D does not decrease the requirements for calcium and phosphorus.

2. In adequate amounts it prevents rickets in children, provided that there is also enough calcium and phosphorus in the diet. In rickets the bones become pliable, and deformities such as bowlegs and knockknees occur when the child begins to walk. The long bones of arms and legs are usually the ones most affected, and a roentgenogram (x-ray picture) will show incomplete calcification on the ends of these bones. Profuse sweating and restlessness are early symptoms of rickets in infants. However, growth may not be retarded, and the infant may outwardly appear to be in perfect health, but when he starts to walk, the deficiency will be manifested. The same deficiency usually leads to malformation of teeth that are forming in the gums.

Human requirements. The recommended daily allowance is 10 μg. cholecalciferol for all persons up to 18 years of age and 10 to 15 μg. for pregnant and lactating women. An adult does not outgrow the need for vitamin D. However, if a person eats a balanced diet and has general exposure to sunlight, he will surely receive a sufficient amount of vitamin D.

Sources. Small but nutritionally insignificant amounts are present in cream, butter, eggs, and liver. Good sources are fish liver oils, milk enriched with vitamin D, and exposure to sunlight under favorable conditions.

One quart of milk enriched with vitamin D contains 400 I.U. of vitamin D (10 μg. cholecalciferol), which is the recommended daily amount for children of all ages. Milk is a very logical product to which vitamin D can be added because milk is also an excellent source of calcium and phosphorus.

Stability. Vitamin D is very stable in heat, during aging, and in storage.

Vitamin K

Functions. Vitamin K is essential in clotting of the blood since it is necessary to the formation of prothrombin, the clotting agent in blood. This vitamin is often used in the control and prevention of certain types of hemorrhages.

Vitamin K is absorbed more completely if bile salts are also present. Patients in whom the flow of bile to the intestines is reduced usually have blood with low clotting ability. However, if bile salts are given with vitamin K concentrate, the clotting time becomes normal.

Human requirements. For most people the intestinal bacteria normally synthesize a constant supply. As yet there is no general agreement on the amount of vitamin K needed by the body.

Vitamin K is usually given to a mother before delivery and to an infant immediately after birth as a precautionary measure.

Sources. Small amounts of vitamin K are found in green leafy vegetables, pork liver, and soybean and other vegetable oils. The main source, however, is that of intestinal bacteria synthesis. Usually a deficiency in vitamin K is the result of poor absorption.

Stability. Vitamin K is fairly stable, although sensitive to light and irradiation. Thus clinical preparations of vitamin K should be kept in dark bottles.

Vitamin E

Functions. Although exact mechanisms are unclear, recent studies indicate several significant functions of vitamin E in relation to human metabolism:

1. It is an effective antioxidant and as such is being used in commercial products to retard spoilage. It is added to therpeutic forms of vitamin A to protect the vitamin from oxidizing before it is absorbed.

2. It seems to preserve the integrity of red blood cells by protecting them from breakdown of their cell walls. Vitamin E therapy has effectively controlled certain anemias in infants.

3. It may also protect the structure and function of muscle tissue. Various stages and forms of muscle degeneration and lesions have been found in pa-

tients with low plasma vitamin E levels—for example, patients with cystic fibrosis or kwashiorkor.

4. It protects unsaturated essential fatty acids, such as linoleic acid, from oxidative breakdown. The amount of vitamin E required by a person has been directly linked with the amount of polyunsaturated fatty acids in his diet.

Human requirements. Vitamin E is clearly an essential nutrient. In recognition of this fact, the revised dietary allowances of the National Research Council in 1968 made a statement concerning vitamin E requirements for the first time and continued it in the 1979 revisions. The recommended daily allowance in α-tocopherol equivalents) for men is 10 mg. daily, and for women, 8 mg., increased in 10 mg. during pregnancy and 11 mg. during lactation. Children's needs range from 3 to 4 mg. for infants, 5 to 7 mg. for young children, and 8 to 10 mg. for boys and girls 10 to 18 years of age.

Sources. The richest sources of vitamin E are the vegetable oils. It is interesting that they are also the richest sources of polyunsaturated fatty acids, which vitamin E protects. Other food sources include milk, eggs, muscle meats, fish, cereals, and leafy vegetables.

Stability. Vitamin E is stable to heat and also to acids, but not to alkalis. It is insoluble in water.

WATER-SOLUBLE VITAMINS
Vitamin C (ascorbic acid)

Functions. Vitamin C performs or assists in the performance of the following body functions:

1. It is essential in the formation and maintenance of the capillary walls.

2. It is essential in the normal healing of wounds and is frequently given following surgical procedures.

3. It prevents the tendency to bleed easily. Pinpoint hemorrhages under the skin, which show up as black-and-blue spots, indicate a lack of vitamin C.

4. It prevents scurvy, which is due to an extreme deficiency of vitamin C. The symptoms are loss of appetite, skin tender to touch, sore mouth with bleeding gums and loosened teeth, black-and-blue spots on the skin, and tenderness of the knee joints.

5. It aids in cementing body cells together and in strengthening the walls of the blood vessels.

6. It helps to guard against infection by stimulating the white blood cells.

7. It is necessary in forming new tissue and regenerating existing tissue.

8. It is implicated in preventing fatigue since lack of ascorbic acid results in the extreme fatigue that occurs after strenuous exercise.

9. It increases the amount of iron absorbed when food is ingested simultaneously.

Human requirements. Vitamin C recommendations were changed in the National Research Council's 1979 revisions. The optimum requirements are 60 mg. for the average man and woman. In women the need is 80 mg. during pregnancy and 100 mg. during lactation.

For children and adolescents the requirements are as follows:

Infants to 1 yr.	35 mg.
1 to 10 yr.	45 mg.
11 to 14 yr.	50 mg.
15 to 18 yr.	60 mg.

Sources. The best sources are citrus fruits. Additional sources include tomatoes, cabbage and other raw leafy vegetables, strawberries, melons, and potatoes. Potatoes are not so high in vitamin C as some of the other sources, but because of the quantity in which they are consumed, they serve as a valuable source.

Stability. Vitamin C is easily destroyed by heat and exposure to air. Because an alkaline medium is very destructive to vitamin C, soda should never be added to food when it is cooked. Acid fruits and vegetables retain their vitamin C content more completely than nonacid fruits and vegetables.

Vitamin C is very soluble in water; therefore, only small amounts of water should be used for cooking. Vegetables should not be cut into small pieces until one is ready to cook them, because the more surface exposed to air, the greater is the destruction of vitamin C.

Thiamin

Functions. Thiamin performs or assists in the performance of the following body functions:

1. It is essential in maintaining good muscle tone, good nerves, and good function of the digestive system. Lack of adequate thiamin is usually accompanied by diminished gastric secretion.

2. It is essential in the metabolism of carbohydrates in the body. The amount of thiamin that is needed is in proportion to the amount of calories consumed; 0.5 mg. for each 1,000 calories is considered adequate. Therefore, in the diet of an average man, 1.5 mg of thiamin would be adequate for a 3,000-calorie diet.

3. It prevents beriberi, which is the manifestation of a severe deficiency of thiamin.

4. It helps maintain a healthy appetite and general well-being. A mild deficiency may cause loss of appetite, certain forms of constipation, poor muscular tone of the intestines, fatigue, and irritability.

Human requirements. The Food and Nutrition Board recommends 1.2 to 1.5 mg. for men and 1 to 1.1 mg. for the average woman, increased during pregnancy and lactation to 1.4 to 1.6 mg.

Men doing hard physical work especially need the optimum amount of thiamin daily, or they will show physical exhaustion.

The recommended amounts for children are as follows:

Infants
    Birth to 6 mo.   0.3 mg.
    6 mo. to 1 yr.   0.5 mg.
Children
    1 to 3 yr.   0.7 mg.
    4 to 6 yr.   0.9 mg.
    6 to 10 yr.   1.2 mg.
    Boys 11 to 14 yr.   1.4 mg.
    Girls 11 to 14 yr.   1.1 mg.
    Boys 15 to 18 yr.   1.4 mg.
    Girls 15 to 18 yr.   1.1 mg.

Sources. Thiamin is present in wheat germ, pork, liver and other organ meats, enriched or whole-grain bread and cereals, and potatoes.

Stability. Thiamin is destroyed by prolonged heating at a high temperature. An alkaline medium is also destructive to thiamin. Thiamin is very soluble in water; therefore, small amounts of water should be used in cooking vegetables. Thiamin in cooked cereals is retained because the water is retained with the cereal.

Riboflavin (vitamin B$_2$)

Functions. Riboflavin is a part of the following body functions:

1. It plays a part in maintaining healthy eyes. A deficiency causes itching and burning of the eyes, sensitivity to light, and headaches.

2. It forms a part of certain enzymes.

3. It is active in maintaining the color and structural tissue of the lips. A deficiency causes the lips to be pale and to split at the corners of the mouth.

4. It is essential to growth.

Human requirements. The Food and Nutrition Board recommends 1.6 mg. for men and 1.2 mg. for the average woman. In women the intake should be increased to 1.5 mg. during pregnancy and to 1.7 mg. during lactation.

The recommended amounts for infants and children are as follows:

Infants
    Birth to 6 mo.   0.4 mg.
    6 mo. to 1 yr.   0.6 mg.
Children
    1 to 3 yr.   0.8 mg.
    4 to 6 yr.   1.0 mg.
    7 to 10 yr.   1.4 mg.
    Boys 11 to 14 yr.   1.6 mg.
    Girls 11 to 14 yr.   1.3 mg.
    Boys 15 to 18 yr.   1.7 mg.
    Girls 15 to 18 yr.   1.3 mg.

Sources. The most important source of riboflavin is milk. Each quart contains 2 mg. Other sources include organ meats, green leafy vegetables, eggs, enriched bread, and cereals.

Stability. Riboflavin in solution, such as in milk, is rapidly destroyed by light. Milk should not be left outside after delivery unless it is in a dark bottle or paper container. Moreover, for obvious reasons, milk should be refrigerated promptly.

Niacin (nicotinic acid)

Functions. Niacin performs or assists in the performance of the following body functions:

1. It forms a part of certain enzymes.

2. It is essential to growth and to the metabolism of carbohydrates.

3. It is necessary to the normal function of the digestive tract and the nervous system.

4. It prevents pellagra, which is manifested by dermatitis, diarrhea, dementia, weakness, vertigo, and anorexia. Before the practice of cereal enrichment began, pellegra occurred most frequently among underprivileged persons in southern states where the diet consisted largely of cornmeal, molasses, and salt pork. When therapeutic doses of niacin and a balanced diet are given, the pellagra clears up.

Human requirements. The amount recommended by the Food and Nutrition Board is 16 to 19 mg. niacin equivalents for men and 13 to 14 mg. for the average woman, increased to 15 or 16 mg. during pregnancy and to 18 or 19 mg. during lactation.

The recommended amounts for infants and children are as follows:

Infants	
Birth to 6 mo.	6 mg.
6 mo. to 1 yr.	8 mg.
Children	
1 to 3 yr.	9 mg.
4 to 6 yr.	11 mg.
7 to 10 yr.	16 mg.
Boys 11 to 14 yr.	18 mg.
Girls 11 to 14 yr.	15 mg.
Boys 15 to 18 yr.	18 mg.
Girls 15 to 18 yr.	14 mg.

Sources. Niacin is present largely in meat, poultry, fish, peanut butter, brown rice, and whole-grain breads and cereals. Niacin is also formed from the amino acid tryptophan. Sixty milligrams of tryptophan equals 1 mg. of niacin. Thus, this amount of tryptophan is called a niacin equivalent.

Stability. Niacin is unusually stable and withstands both heat and contact with oxygen. However, it is soluble in water, and large amounts of niacin may be discarded with the water in which vegetables are cooked.

Folacin (folic acid)

Functions. Folic acid assists in the performance of the following body functions:

1. It is essential in the formation of all body cells, especially the red blood cells.

2. It contributes to the successful treatment of certain types of anemia when used in combination with vitamin B_{12}.

Human requirements. In its 1968 revisions, the National Research Council made a statement for the first time about folacin requirements and continued it in the current revisions. The daily allowance for adults is 400 μg. During pregnancy this is raised to 800 μg. daily, and for lactation to 500 μg. Requirements for children range from 30 μg. daily for infants to 400 μg. daily for adolescents.

Sources. The main sources of folic acid are liver, meats, fish, nuts, yeast, green vegetables, legumes, eggs, whole grains, and mushrooms.

Stability. Storage and cooking losses are quite high, regardless of the method of cooking used.

Pantothenic acid

Functions. Pantothenic acid assists in the performance of the following body functions:

1. It is involved in the metabolism of carbohydrates.

2. It is essential in the synthesis and breakdown of fatty acids, sterols, and steroid hormones.

Human requirements. The amount of pantothenic acid necessary for human beings has not yet been determined.

Sources. Pantothenic acid is present in most ordinary food, therefore, there should be no deficiency in the average normal diet. Liver, meat, cereal, and milk are reliable sources. A diet of 2,500 calories selected from both animal and plant foods would provide approximately 10 mg. a day.

Stability. Pantothenic acid is stable in heat but is water-soluble and sensitive to alkalis.

Vitamin B_{12}

Function. Vitamin B_{12} is the extrinsic factor involved in the treatment of pernicious anemia. When administered parenterally, it relieves the many symptoms of pernicious anemia.

Human requirements. For the first time, the 1968 revisions of the National Research Council also included daily allowances for vitamin B_{12} and continued them in the current revisions. The council recommends 3 mg. daily for adults, with increases for pregnant and lactating women to 4 mg. Requirements for children range from 0.5 mg. for infants to 3 mg. for adolescents.

Sources. Liver, kidney, and fresh muscle meats are the richest known sources at the present time.

Stability. Since vitamin B_{12} occurs as a protein complex in foods (hence, mainly in foods of animal origin), it is stable in ordinary cooking processes.

Pyridoxine (vitamin B_6)

Functions. The following body functions are performed by pyridoxine:
1. It is involved in the conversion of tryptophan to niacin.
2. It helps to prevent muscular weakness and certain nervous disorders.
3. It aids in various interconversions of amino acids.
4. It supplies increased metabolic demands during pregnancy.

Human requirements. For the first time, in its 1968 recommended allowances the National Research Council made a statement concerning pyridoxine requirements and continued it in the current revisions. The recommendation for adults is 2 mg. per day for women and 2.2 mg. for men to assure a margin of safety for variances in individual needs. Children's needs range progressively from 0.3 mg. for infants to 1.8 mg. for adolescents.

Sources. It occurs freely in many different foods, including pork, glandular meats, lamb, and veal. Lesser amounts are found in fish, beef, legumes, potatoes, oatmeal, bananas, cabbage, and carrots.

Stability. Pyridoxine is stable in heat but it is soluble in water and is sensitive to light and alkalis.

SUMMARY

The average healthy adult requires vitamins but does not require vitamin supplements. Vitamins are best purchased at the grocery counter in foods that supply the variety of nutrients needed by the body. A well-balanced diet will provide ample vitamins for usual needs. Therefore, the use of supplementary vitamins in addition to an adequate diet is rarely necessary; it is expensive, and in some cases, it is dangerous. Vitamins A and D can both be toxic in excessive doses.

Vitamin D taken in excess may cause anorexia, nausea, vomiting, diarrhea, weakness, and weight loss. Also, an excess of calcium may be deposited in the body. An adequate diet should give enough vitamin A for normal persons. Evidence concerning the toxicity of an excess of vitamin A emphasizes the need for caution in the use of vitamin A and D preparations. Some of the signs of vitamin A toxicity are skin lesions, thinning hair, coarse skin, and often pains in the joints.

The other vitamins are not toxic, but if an excess is taken, it is simply excreted, hence wasted.

Vitamins are essential, but clinical preparations of them should be reserved for states of debilitation, malnutrition, and clinical disease.

Questions on vitamins

1. What are the functions of vitamins in the body?
2. Name the six vitamins that the body must receive daily.
3. How were vitamins first discovered?
4. What are the fat-soluble vitamins?
5. What are the water-soluble vitamins?
6. What is meant by deficiencies?
7. What is meant by subclinical deficiencies?
8. Which vitamins are we able to store to any extent?
9. What are the functions of vitamin A?
10. What is the adult requirement of vitamin A?
11. Name some good sources of vitamin A.
12. Name some good sources of carotene.
13. Compare the vitamin value of carotene and of true vitamin A.
14. Discuss the stability of vitamin A.
15. How is a deficiency in vitamin A manifested?
16. What are the functions of vitamin D?
17. Does vitamin D decrease the requirement of calcium and phosphorus?
18. What parts of the body are usually most affected by rickets?
19. What is the average daily requirement of vitamin D?
20. What are the sources of vitamin D?
21. What is one source of vitamin D that will provide an adequate daily intake?
22. Is vitamin D stable?
23. How is a deficiency in vitamin D manifested?
24. What is the function of vitamin K?
25. How does bile affect the absorption of vitamin K?
26. What are the sources of vitamin K?
27. When is vitamin K therapy sometimes used?
28. What are the food sources of vitamin K?
29. What are the functions of vitamin C?
30. What is the daily requirement of vitamin C for adults?
31. What are the food sources of vitamin C?
32. Discuss the stability of vitamin C.
33. How is a deficiency in vitamin C manifested?
34. What are the functions of thiamin?
35. What is the average adult requirement of thiamin?
36. When is it necessary to increase the intake of thiamin?
37. What are some good food sources of thiamin?
38. Discuss the stability of thiamin.
39. What are the results of a deficiency in thiamin?
40. What are the functions of riboflavin?
41. What is the average adult requirement of riboflavin?
42. What are the best food sources of riboflavin?
43. Discuss the stability of riboflavin.
44. What are the results of a deficiency in riboflavin?
45. What are the functions of niacin?
46. What is the average adult requirement of niacin?
47. What are the best food sources of niacin?
48. What are the functions of folic acid?
49. What are the functions of pantothenic acid, and what are its best sources?

50. What is the function of vitamin B_{12}, and what are its best sources?
51. What vitamins are toxic if taken in excessive amounts?
52. What occurs if an excess of the other vitamins is taken?

Suggestions for additional study

1. Prepare a chart showing the principal functions, sources, and requirements of each of the vitamins discussed in this chapter.
2. On one page of your notebook put illustrations of foods that will give an adequate supply of these vitamins for one day.
3. Prepare a report on the work of Dr. Joseph Goldberger in his search for the cause of pellagra.

References

Church, C. F., and Church, H. N.: Food values of portions commonly used, ed. 11, Philadelphia, 1970, J. B. Lippincott Co.

Guthrie, H. A.: Introductory nutrition, ed. 4, St. Louis, 1979, The C. V. Mosby Co.

Williams, S. R.: Nutrition and diet therapy, ed. 3, St. Louis, 1977, The C. V. Mosby Co.

Williams, S. R.: Essentials of nutrition and diet therapy, ed. 2, St. Louis, 1978, The C. V. Mosby Co.

8

Digestion

Digestion is the process by which food is broken up in the gastrointestinal tract and made ready for absorption in the body. All food must be absorbed into the bloodstream before it can be used by the body. Before food can enter the bloodstream, it must go through a series of mechanical and chemical changes that constitute digestion. The chemical changes are brought about by the action of enzymes. Enzymes are organic protein substances that accelerate the various processes in both plant and animal tissues without having their own composition changed in these processes. They are responsible for bringing about the process of breaking the food down into simpler forms that can enter the blood. Enzyme action is specific—that is, a particular enzyme will act only on a particular class of foodstuff and will produce no action on any other. Enzymes usually receive their name from the substance on which they act. For example, sucrase acts only on sucrose.

FOOD CHANGES IN THE MOUTH

The actions in the mouth are both chemical and mechanical. The first change in food occurs during the process of chewing, when the food is broken up into small bits by the process of mastication and is softened and moistened by the saliva, which prepares the food for swallowing. Muscles at the base of the tongue are responsible for the process of swallowing.

The chemical change in the mouth occurs when ptyalin, the enzyme secreted by the saliva, acts on starch. However, food usually stays in the mouth too short a period of time for any significant chemical breakdown of starch to occur.

After the food leaves the mouth, it passes quickly through the esophagus to the stomach, partly by gravity and partly by muscular action.

DIGESTION IN THE STOMACH

The three areas of the stomach are the fundus; the body, or middle portion; and the pylorus, or small end. The fundus, or upper part of the stomach, receives the food mass first. The amount of the food mass is gradually reduced as

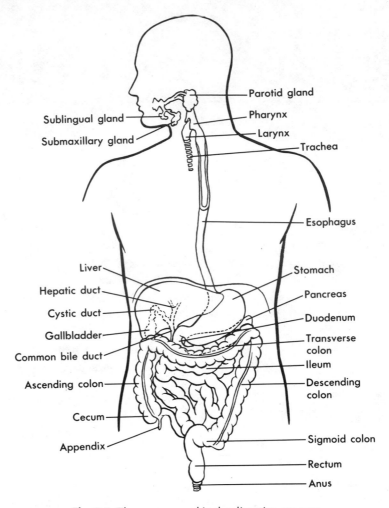

Fig. 7-1. The organs used in the digestive process.

small portions move into the middle area of the stomach, where the secretion of gastric juice occurs and gastric digestion proceeds. From 2 to $2^{1}/_{2}$ quarts of gastric juice are secreted daily. It contains hydrochloric acid and the enzymes pepsin, rennin, and gastric lipase. Pepsin acts on proteins, changing them to simpler forms. Rennin brings about the curdling of milk and acts on casein, one of the proteins in milk. The gastric lipase breaks down the emulsified fats, such as those in egg yolk and cream. It does not act on the fats of meat, which are not emulsified. The food mass, which is by this time semiliquid, moves toward the pyloric end of the stomach and into the intestines by means of peristaltic waves, which are rhythmic contractions of the stomach.

Food remains in the stomach for varying lengths of time, depending on the type of food. Carbohydrates leave the stomach very quickly, and protein leaves more quickly than fat. Small amounts of food leave the stomach in less time than a large meal.

DIGESTION IN THE SMALL INTESTINE

When the food is thoroughly mixed with the gastric juice, the pylorus, which is a strong sphincter muscle, opens, or, more often, peristaltic waves increase in intensity and force the semifluid food, called chyme, into the duodenum. The presence of acid in the chyme causes the mucous membrane of the intestine to secrete a substance called secretin, which in turn causes the pancreas to send pancreatic juice into the duodenum.

In the small intestine the food is acted on by the pancreatic juice, by bile, which is secreted by the liver and then concentrated and stored in the gallbladder for release as needed to emulsify fats, and by the intestinal juice—all of which act in unison. These juices are alkaline, and their first action is to neutralize the hydrochloric acid remaining in the food mass coming from the stomach.

The pancreatic juice has five enzymes: one that acts on starch, even raw starch; three that work in sequence to help complete the digestion of proteins; and another that completes enough initial digestion of fats to prepare them for absorption. The final digestion of fats takes place inside the intestinal walls by an enteric fat enzyme secreted in these cells during absorption.

Among the enzymes in the intestinal juice are two that complete protein digestion and a set of three that complete the breakdown of carbohydrates to simple sugars. The bile secreted by the liver aids in the digestion of fats by emulsifying the fats so that the pancreatic juice can come more readily into contact with the fat particles.

In summary of the digestive processes, the digestion of starch begins slightly in the mouth and is brought to completion in the small intestine. The digestion of sugars takes place in the small intestine. The digestion of emulsified fat may begin in the stomach and be carried to completion in the small intestine, but the digestion of other fats take place almost wholly in the intestine. The digestion of protein begins in the stomach and is brought to completion in the small intestine.

ABSORPTION OF FOOD

No absorption of food nutrients takes place in the mouth or stomach, although water is absorbed to some extent. Practically all the nutrients are absorbed from the small intestine, and a small amount is sometimes absorbed from the large intestine. Vitamins and minerals are absorbed from the small intestine, along with carbohydrates, proteins, and fats.

The inside of the small intestine is lined with fingerlike projections called villi. These villi greatly increase the absorbing surface of the intestine. Each villus has many small capillaries, an artery, and a vein, and in the center of each is a lymph vessel called a lacteal.

The end products in the digestion of protein are the amino acids, and the end product in the digestion of carbohydrate is glucose. These products pass through the villi in the intestinal walls and enter directly into the bloodstream. The end products of the digestion of fat, fatty acids and glycerides, are absorbed through the lacteals in the villi and thence through the lymphatic system, finally entering the portal blood system to the liver.

When digestion has been completed in the small intestine, what remains of the fluid mass passes on into the large intestine, where further absorption of fluid takes place.

FOOD CHANGES IN THE LARGE INTESTINE

Although the large intestine does not secrete any enzymes, digestion may continue by means of the digestive juices carried into it with the food. There is some absorption of food material from part of the large intestine. The indigestible fiber materials, with some digestive juices, bacteria, and cellular debris of the body tissues, pass out of the body as feces.

Fiber, or cellulose, is found in all whole grains, vegetables, and fruits. It influences transit time and rate of absorption, and it produces bulk in the intestines with a laxative effect in the colon.

Water is essential to the operation of all the cells of the body. It is contained both within the cells and in the fluids that surround the cells. Some of the functions of water are as follows:

1. Essential constituent of all tissues and fluids of the body.
2. Essential in transporting all nutrients from the digestive tract into the bloodstream and from one cell to another
3. Essential in regulating body temperature
4. Excretion of waste products in solution through the kidneys and bowels
5. Lubrication of the joints and moistening of the viscera for easier movement in the abdominal cavity

Six to eight glasses of fluid in some form should be taken daily. Many of our foods, especially some of the fruits and vegetables, contain large amounts of water.

Water is reused in the body time and again. Humans can live longer without food than without water. Max Rubner, the German physiologist, has stated that we can lose all of our reserve glycogen, all of our reserve fat, and about half of our body protein and still survive, but a 10% loss of water is serious, and a 20% to 22% loss is fatal.

FACTORS AFFECTING DIGESTION

Digestibility, the ease and rapidity of digestion, is affected by a number of conditions.

Finely divided foods—mashed, ground, or pureed—are more easily digested. The same result may be achieved by thorough chewing, except in the case of pureed food. Liquid foods are absorbed more quickly than solid ones. The amount of food taken at one time has an influence on the ease and rapidity of digestion. Therefore, it is important that persons who are acutely ill have small feedings at frequent intervals to facilitate ease of digestion.

Excessive peristalsis may occur in the intestines if there is inflammation or infection, resulting in diarrhea. Constipation may result from sluggish peristalsis.

Some of the causes of indigestion are as follows:

1. Improper selection of food (Too much fat in the diet will inhibit the secretion of the gastric juice and thereby delay digestion. Concentrated sweets may irritate the digestive tract. Gas-forming fruits and vegetables may be difficult to digest. Acids and spices may cause discomfort by increasing the acidity of the gastric contents.)
2. Overeating, which overtaxes the digestive system
3. Undereating
4. Eating too fast, which results in swallowing food that is only half chewed
5. Food to which one is not accustomed (especially if the food is not served attractively)
6. Food poorly prepared (Included are fried foods that are cooked at too low a temperature, with the result that too much fat is absorbed by the food. Likewise, overheated fats are irritating to the stomach.)
7. Eating when too tired
8. Eating when mentally disturbed or emotionally upset
9. Lack of exercise
10. Excessive use of alcoholic beverages

SATIETY VALUE OF FOODS

The satiety value of a food can be measured by the length of time the food remains in the stomach and by the amount of gastric juice stimulated by it. *Meat* is first in satiety value because it calls forth great physiological activity in the stomach. It is a well-known saying that a meal containing meat "sticks to the ribs." Next to meat in satiety value is *milk*. The richer the milk, the greater its satiety value. *Eggs* are likewise very satisfying. Raw eggs leave the stomach sooner than soft-boiled eggs, and hard-boiled eggs remain the longest. Cooked eggs are also more easily digested than raw eggs. *Fish* is of lower satiety value than meat or eggs. *Bread* may be less desired unless it is buttered. *Potatoes* belong in the same group as bread. *Green vegetables* have relatively low satisfying qualities. *Fats* in general increase the satiety of a meal by retarding the emptying of the stomach.

The sight of a properly set table that contains attractive food is very appealing, but if the same food is poorly prepared and poorly served, it is very unappealing.

Questions on digestion

1. What is digestion?
2. What do enzymes do in the digestive process?
3. What is meant by the specific action of enzymes?
4. What is the most active enzyme in saliva?
5. What changes in the food takes place in the mouth?
6. What happens to the food in the fundus part of the stomach?
7. What are the active ingredients of gastric juice?
8. Discuss the emptying rate of various food nutrients from the stomach.
9. What are the juices that act on food in the intestine?
10. Where does most of the absorption of food take place?
11. What is the function of the villi?
12. What products of digestion pass into the blood?
13. What products of digestion pass into the lymphatic system?
14. Where are are the minerals and vitamins absorbed?
15. Does the large intestine secrete any enzymes?
16. What factors affect the ease of digestion?
17. How much water or other liquid should be drunk daily?
18. What are the functions of water in the body?
19. What are some of the causes of indigestion?
20. What is meant by satiety value?
21. List six foods in the order of their satiety value.

Suggestion for additional study

1. If possible, secure a film showing the various processes involved in the digestion of food.

References

Guthrie, H. A.: Introductory nutrition, ed. 4, St. Louis, 1979, The C. V. Mosby Co.

Williams, S. R.:Nutrition and diet therapy, ed. 3, St. Louis, 1977, The C. V. Mosby Co.

Williams, S. R.: Essentials of nutrition and diet therapy, ed. 2, St. Louis, 1978, The C. V. Mosby Co.

PART TWO

COMMUNITY NUTRITION
the life cycle

9

Nutrition for the various age groups

NUTRITION FOR CHILDREN
Infancy

Almost any mother can breast-feed her baby if she has had the proper diet during pregnancy and if she maintains that diet during the time she wants to nurse the baby. Human milk provides the ideal first food for the human infant and is the primary recommendation of pediatricians and nutritionists alike. Its content of nutrients is uniquely adapted to meet the growth needs of the infant. Moreover, the form of these materials in human milk is better utilized by the baby than are those corresponding constituents of cow's milk. There is more iron in human milk, which is likewise better absorbed and utilized by the baby. Human milk contains more vitamins A and K, ascorbic acid, and niacin. It also gives the infant immunity to certain diseases.

Breast-feeding gives the baby a good start in life. It may be especially important during the first month. It also helps the mother's uterus to return to normal more quickly. It assists in the important early "bonding" process, building a warm and affectionate relationship between mother and child.

The infant may be weaned from breast-feeding after the sixth month, unless another pregnancy or an illness of the mother occurs sooner. The average age for weaning the baby under usual circumstances is about 9 months.

Infants will more or less establish their own rate of weight gain. As long as they make a steady gain in weight and appear to be satisfied, one can assume that they are getting enough to eat.

During the first 6 months babies will usually make an average gain of 6 ounces a week. They should have doubled their birth weight by the time they are 6 months of age. The gain in weight is slower during the second 6 months, but most babies triple their birth weight by the time they are 1 year of age. Of course, there are variations to this that are perfectly normal.

Feeding schedules should be elastic to a degree, although there should be an attempt to have a reasonably regular schedule. Usually the feedings will be about 3 hours apart at first and, later, 4 hours apart. The 2 A.M. feeding can usually be omitted after the first 2 months, and after the first 5 months the 10 P.M. one will no longer be needed. If for some reason, however, the mother finds breast-feeding inappropriate to her situation, she may choose bottle-feeding as an alternative, using a home-prepared or commercial formula, usually made from cow's milk.

The milk most generally used in home-prepared infant formulas is canned evaporated milk. Other types of milk that are used are fresh, pasteurized, homogenized milk, dry milk, lactic acid milk, and goat's milk. When the infant is allergic to cow's milk, soybean milk is sometimes used with good results. If canned or dried milk is used, it must be refrigerated after the can or package is opened.

Cow's milk is higher in protein, fat, and most minerals and lower in sugar than human milk. For this reason, water and sugar are added to cow's milk in making a formula. Sugar is usually added in the form of corn syrup or Dextri-maltose. Most of the calories required by the infant are supplied by the milk itself; the additional needed calories are supplied by the sugar. Water is added to dilute the protein and to meet the fluid requirements of the infant, which are 75 ml. per pound of body weight.

Babies require more protein per pound of body weight than adults. Whereas the adult's protein needs are 0.4 gram per pound, those of the baby are 0.9 to 1.4 grams of protein in human milk or 1.4 to 1.9 grams of protein in cow's milk per pound of body weight. The protein of human milk is better adapted to the needs of the infant than the protein of cow's milk.

A baby also requires more calories per pound than an adult, the requirement being 54 calories per pound from 1 to 3 months of age, 50 calories per pound from 4 to 9 months of age, and 45 calories per pound from 10 to 12 months of age, whereas the adult requires only 18 to 20 calories per pound. The infant needs more calories because he has more body surface in proportion to his weight and because of growth and activity.

In calculating the formula for an infant, one must consider the calories and the amount of protein needed, as well as the amount of fluids the infant should have.

As an example, a formula for a 14-pound baby, 5 months of age, is calculated as follows:

Number of feedings: 5 (if at 4-hour intervals)
Size of feedings: 7 oz.
Daily total: 5 times 7 oz. equals 35 oz.
Whole milk: 14 times 1.75 oz. equals 24.5 oz.
Water: 35 minus 24.5 equals 10.5 oz.
Sugar: 1 oz.

This formula contains 24.5 grams of protein, or 1.7 grams for each pound of body weight.

A baby will probably be given vitamin supplements as early as 1 week of age. The dosage will depend on the vitamin preparation being used and the pediatrician's prescription for the individual baby's needs. Breast milk from a healthy mother who has had a good diet meets the nutritional requirements of the infant for the first 6 months. It is currently recommended by pediatricians

Table 9-1. Guideline for addition of solid foods to infant's diet during the first year*

When to start	Foods added	Feeding
First month	Vitamins A, D, and C in multivitamin preparation (according to prescription)	Once daily at a feeding time
Fifth to sixth month, in gradual small additions	Cereal and strained cooked fruit Egg yolk (at first hard-boiled and sieved, later soft-boiled or poached)	10 A.M. and 6 P.M.
	Strained, cooked vegetable and meat	2 P.M.
	Zwieback or hard toast	At any feeding
Seventh to ninth month	Meat: beef, lamb, or liver (broiled or baked and finely chopped) Potato: baked or boiled, and mashed or sieved	10 A.M. or 6 P.M.

Suggested meal plan for age 8 months to 1 year or older		
7 A.M.	Milk	8 oz.
	Cereal	2 to 3 tbs.
	Strained fruit	2 to 3 tbs.
	Zwieback or dry toast	
Noon	Milk	8 oz.
	Vegetables	2 to 3 tbs.
	Chopped meat or one whole egg	
	Puddings or cooked fruit	2 to 3 tbs.
3 P.M.	Milk	4 oz.
	Toast, zwieback, or crackers	
6 P.M.	Milk	8 oz.
	Whole egg or chopped meat	
	Potato, baked or mashed	2 tbs.
	Pudding or cooked fruit	2 to 3 tbs.
	Zwieback or toast	

*Semisolid foods should be given immediately after breast- or bottle-feeding. One or 2 teaspoons should be given at first. If food is accepted and tolerated well, amount should be increased to 1 to 2 tablespoons per feeding.

Note: Banana may be substituted for fruit and cottage cheese for meat or egg in any meal.

and nutritionists that solid foods not be added to the baby's diet until 5 or 6 months of age. The infant's system cannot utilize them very well before then, they are not needed yet, and more often they lay the foundation for infant and childhood obesity patterns from overeating.

The premature baby requires special care. The stomach is smaller than that of the normal baby, and the digestive system is less developed. The fluid requirements of the premature baby are higher than those of the normal baby. The premature baby does not tolerate fats very well. He needs more calcium and more protein than the full-term baby because almost 50% of the calcium and phosphorus is deposited during the last month of pregnancy. The premature baby, however, does better on a formula of cow's milk (usually low or nonfat because of poor fat tolerance) than on human milk because cow's milk is higher in calcium and protein. The cow's milk formula may be supplemented by human milk if the mother desires. She may express the milk by hand or with a common hand breast pump and then give it to the baby by bottle until he is strong enough to suck well. The bottle nipple should be soft with larger-than-usual holes.

Table 9-1 is a summary of the additions that may be made to the formula or to a breast-feeding for the normal full-term baby.

Above all, the meal hour should be a happy time. The attitude toward the meal hour, either happy or unhappy, will carry over into the later years of a child's life.

Preschool children

During the latent growth period of childhood, the growth rate is slower and more erratic than that of infancy, and the child's appetite and food intake will vary accordingly. A variety of foods should be offered to the child, with an avoidance of too many refined sweets.

During the preschool years the child begins to eat an increasing variety of foods served to the rest of the family. The child at this age likes food that he can eat with his hands, such as raw carrot sticks and chicken drumsticks. His meat should be cut in bite-sized pieces, and he may have vegetables and raw fruits regularly.

Foods should be served attractively and in small amounts. If the child wants more, he may have a second serving. Servings of food that are too large discourage a child from eating. Introduce a new food in small portions and at a time when the child is hungry. If he refuses it, simply try it again in a few days. Do not bribe or coax the child to eat. He will only repeat the performance to gain more attention.

Schoolchildren (5 to 12 years)

New problems arise when the child starts to school. If he is not awakened early enough in the morning, he may not have time to eat a good breakfast without hurrying or worrying that he is going to be late. Association with other children who do not have good nutritional habits may cause the child to question his own routine.

The schoolchild usually has a good appetite. Meals should be kept simple but adequate. The best way to influence children to establish good nutritional habits is for the parents to set a good example by eating the correct foods themselves.

Good mental development goes hand in hand with good nutrition. The child who is well nourished will be more alert in the classroom than the malnourished child.

The school-lunch program has helped somewhat to improve nutrition, especially of children in underprivileged areas.

The adolescent

Many adolescents eat a less well-balanced diet than persons in any other age group except possibly elderly persons. Teenagers, for the most part, choose their own food. The consumption of soft drinks, hot dogs, and candy bars often reduces the intake of milk and other valuable foods. The adolescent is at an age when it is important to conform to his friends in eating habits as well as in the social amenities.

Boys of this age usually eat a sufficient amount of food but not always the right kind. Girls are inclined to eat less than they need because of their desire to keep thin. If they are little overweight, they may try to reduce in a foolish manner. Poor food selection is responsible for much of the overweight among teenage girls. Overweight girls can learn that they may eat a balanced diet and at the same time reduce safely.

Teenage girls may not realize that good looks and good nutrition go together. Moreover, many girls marry while still in their teens, and with a background of an inadequate diet, they are very poorly prepared for the demands of pregnancy. These girls must complete their own growth and development and at the same time supply the extra needs of the baby. It is necessary to have a very carefully planned diet to accomplish this. A teenage girl who is poorly prepared nutritionally for pregnancy will no doubt experience more of the complications incident to pregnancy, such as toxemia, abortion, premature labor, and eclampsia. A girl who has maintained good nutrition throughout her teenage years and who continues a well-balanced diet throughout pregnancy will no doubt deliver a normal, healthy, full-term infant.

NUTRITION FOR ADULTS

Both heredity and nutrition are major factors in determining the length of normal lives.

An adult should, during his younger adult years, give optimum care to his body. We do not expect a car to run for years without any care; yet many people seem to expect their bodies to do just that. The organs and tissues of the body do their respective jobs for many years if they are well nourished and protected. By giving the body intelligent care, a person can have a much healthier and more satisfying old age. The signs of old age may be postponed, but one cannot expect to wait until old age to give the body scientific care. Good nutrition is only one of the health practices that help to maintain health and vigor, but it is one that can be practiced more readily and yet is abused more frequently than any other.

Life expectancy has increased from 47 years in 1900 to about 77 years currently because of modern science. Much of this increase is due to better prenatal and infant care, better care of chronic diseases of middle-aged and older persons, and more complete control of infectious and communicable diseases.

In addition to prolonging life, modern scientific health care has resulted in a definite increase in the years of usefulness during middle age and a postponement of the diseases incident to old age.

A person may have either too much or too little food, or he may make the wrong choice of food. Eating too much food seems to present a problem for some persons in the United States, and obesity results. For others, however, caught in the morass of poverty, food is scare or at times nonexistent, and hunger or malnutrition results. Weight should be watched carefully and a deviation of 10% to 15% above or below the normal weight should be investigated.

When watching calories, one should choose them wisely. A person on a limited financial budget is careful to spend each dollar to good advantage, and the same should hold true for a person who is on a limited caloric budget. Adequate proteins, minerals, and vitamins are as important in a reducing diet as in a normal one, even though it is more difficult on a reducing diet to secure the protective foods in adequate amounts.

Vitamin preparations are usually not needed by the healthy adult. If a person eats a balanced diet, he will usually receive sufficient vitamins.

During pregnancy

It is very important to the health of both mother and child that a prospective mother eat a well-balanced diet with increased amounts of all the essential nutrients. The woman who has always eaten a well-balanced diet has a better chance of having a healthy baby and of remaining in good health herself than the woman who has been undernourished.

A report by the National Research Council has established important changes in the nutritional care provided for women during pregancy.* Contrary

---

*National Research Council: Maternal nutrition and the course of pregnancy, Washington, D.C., 1970, National Academy of Sciences.

to prior belief, weight should *not* be restricted during pregnancy nor should salt be restricted. Studies indicate that women deliver healthy babies over a wide range of weight gain; it is not the *amount* of weight gain but the *quality* of that weight gain and the *quality* of the diet the woman eats to produce the gain that determines the health of the baby and the mother.

The average weight of the products of a normal pregnancy are given in the following list:

Products	Weight (lb.)
Fetus	7.5
Placenta	1
Amniotic fluid	2
Uterus (increase)	2.5
Breast tissue (increase)	3
Blood volume (increase)	4 (1,500 ml.)
Maternal stores	4 to 8
	24 to 28

It is clearly evident, therefore, that calorie restriction during pregancy is unphysiological and potentially harmful to the developing baby and to the mother. A calorie-restricted diet cannot supply all the increased nutrient demands essential to the growth process going on during pregnancy. This weight reduction should *never* be undertaken during pregnancy. To the contrary, adequate weight gain should be supported with the use of a nourishing, well-balanced diet as outlined in this discussion.

About 2 to 4 pounds is an average weight gain during the first trimester. Thereafter about a pound a week during the remainder of the pregnancy is usual.

Just as with restriction of calories, routine restriction of sodium is unphysiological and unfounded. Physicians who prescribe diets low in calories and salt are placing pregnant women and their offspring at a distinct disadvantage and at an unnecessary risk. A number of studies have indicated the need for sodium during pregnancy and the harm to maternal-fetal health that results from salt restriction. Combined with the added injury of a routine use of diuretics, such a program places the pregnant woman and her baby in double jeopardy. The National Research Council report on "Maternal Nutrition and the Course of Pregnancy" labels such routine use of salt-free diets and diuretics as potentially dangerous.

Instead of a restricted diet approach, the National Research Council emphasizes a positive approach based on an increased demand for key nutrients during pregnancy. The major focus is on *protein*. Protein is the primary need because it is the growth element for body tissues. The new recommended dietary allowances of the National Research Council indicate a need for 80 to 85 grams of protein daily during pregnancy. This amount represents an increase of about 50% over the normal adult diet. Moreover, a large number of high-risk or active pregnant women need even more protein, 80 to 100 grams daily, or about double their previous intake.

A number of reasons for this increased protein need during pregnancy reflect the tremendous growth period involved:

1. *Rapid growth of the baby.* The mere increase in size of the infant from one cell to millions of cells in a 7-pound child indicates how much protein is required for such rapid growth.

2. *Development of the placenta.* The mature placenta requires sufficient protein for its complete development as a vital organ to sustain, support, and nourish the baby during growth.

3. *Growth of maternal tissues.* Increased development of breast and uterine tissue is required to support pregnancy.

4. *Increased maternal circulating blood volume.* The mother's blood volume increases during pregnancy 20% to 50% over her normal volume. This increased amount of circulating blood is necessary to nourish the child and support the increased metabolic work load involved. With this increased amount of blood comes a need for increased synthesis of the components of blood, especially hemoglobin and plasma protein. Both of these substances are proteins vital to the support of the pregnancy. Increased hemoglobin is needed to supply oxygen to the growing cells. Increased plasma protein (albumin) is needed to keep the increased blood volume circulating. Albumin in the blood provides the osmotic force constantly needed to pull the tissue fluids back into circulation after they have bathed and nourished the cells, thus preventing abnormal accumulation of water in the tissues (edema).

5. *Formation of amniotic fluid.* The fluid surrounding the baby is designed to protect him from shock or injury. This fluid contains protein, and hence its formation requires still more protein.

6. *Storage reserves.* Increased tissue storage reserves are needed in the mother's body to prepare for labor, delivery, the immediate postpartum period, and lactation.

The second major focus of the diet during pregnancy is on *calories.* The amount of calories should be sufficient to meet the increased demands for energy and nutrients and to spare protein for the tissue-building requirements listed before. The current revisions of the National Research Council recommend a 15% to 20% increase over the usual intake of calories in an adult woman. Nutritionally deficient women or those more physically active would easily need more. The average need is about 2,400 calories, with some pregnant women requiring more calories. The emphasis should always be a positive one on ample calories to secure the necessary nutrient and energy needs.

The key minerals, calcium and phosphorus, along with vitamin D, are essential for a mother's own body needs and for the bones and teeth of the fetus.

Calcium is also necessary for proper clotting of the blood. A diet that includes 1 quart of milk and generous amounts of green vegetables, whole-grain cereals, and eggs will supply sufficient calcium for the needs of both the mother and the fetus.

Two additional minerals needed in increased amounts during pregnancy are iron and iodine. An adequate supply of iron is essential for the production of hemoglobin and for the necessary prenatal storage of iron in the body of the infant. An intake of iodine is essential to meet the increased thyroid activity associated with the greater need for thyroxine, the hormone controlling the increased basal metabolic rate. This increase of iodine is ensured by the use of iodized salt.

Vitamins are also needed in increased amounts during pregnancy. These include vitamins A and C, important elements in tissue growth, and the B vitamins needed for energy production and protein synthesis. One B vitamin, folic acid, is especially needed to build mature red blood cells. A vitamin and mineral supplement including folic acid is usually used during pregnancy.

Vomiting, which sometimes occurs during the first 3 months of pregnancy, may usually be relieved by one or more of the following dietary changes:

1. A lower intake of fat
2. A dry diet at the meal hour, with fluids between meals
3. An emphasis on foods high in carbohydrate
4. Eating dry toast or crackers on awakening in the morning

Toxemia does not usually occur in women whose diets have been adequate throughout pregnancy. It occurs more frequently when the diet is low in protein and vitamins. A woman who is underweight is more likely to have premature labor and toxemia. When toxemia does occur, it is usually during the last 3 months. The dietary treatment consists of a diet as described in Table 9-2, rich in protein, minerals, and vitamins.

During lactation

There is even greater need for increased nutrients during lactation. A normal baby will require 2 to 2¹/₂ ounces of the mother's milk per pound of body weight. A 7-pound infant will take approximately 18 ounces, and it is easy to understand why additional food is required by the mother. One ounce of breast milk contains 20 calories. The diet of the mother who is breast-feeding her baby should be high in protein and calories, with an increase in fluids. High caloric liquids, especially those made with milk, should be taken between meals, rather than consumed with the meals, in an attempt to consume more of the necessary calories at mealtime. About 6 cups of milk should be used in some from each day.

A summary of foods in a daily plan for pregnancy and lactation is shown in Table 9-2.

Table 9-2. Daily food plan for pregnancy and lactation

Food	Nonpregnant state	Pregnancy	Lactation
Milk (cheese, ice cream, other milk-based foods, skim milk, or buttermilk)	2 cups	4 cups	6 cups
Meat (lean meat, fish, poultry, cheese, occasionally dried beans or peas)	1 serving (3 to 4 oz.)	2 servings (6 to 8 oz.; include liver frequently)	2$\frac{1}{2}$ servings (8 oz.)
Egg	1	1 or 2	1 or 2
Vegetable*: Dark green or deep yellow	1	1	1 or 2
Vitamin C-rich food*: Good sources—citrus fruit, berries, cantaloupe Fair sources—tomatoes, cabbage, greens, potatoes in skin	1 good source or 2 fair sources	1 good source *and* 1 fair source, or 2 good sources	1 good source *and* 1 fair source, or 2 good sources
Other vegetables and fruits	1 serving	2 servings	2 servings
Breads and cereals (Enriched or whole-grain; 1 slice bread = 1 serving)	3 servings	4 or 5 servings	5 servings
Butter or fortified margarine	As desired or needed for calories	As desired or needed for calories	As desired or needed for calories

*Use some raw daily.

NUTRITION FOR THE GERIATRIC PATIENT

Nutrition and metabolism are fundamentally very similar throughout the life-span. Good nutrition is as necessary in later life as in the early years, but the process of aging presents special problems, even as infancy and childhood have their special needs.

Geriatric medicine, to be truly effective, should be largely preventive medicine. A well-balanced diet from 40 to 60 years of age plays a big role in assuring a healthy life from 60 to 80 years of age. We are largely what we are today because of our yesterdays. The older we become, the more yesterdays there are to affect us. Since all persons have varying types of yesterdays, with different problems, older persons become increasingly divergent in their reactions to foods and to life in general.

Some of the following points should be considered in planning diets for members of the older age group:

1. The diet should be well balanced and high in proteins, vitamins, and

minerals. In order to allow for the wastage during diminished absorption, it is well to give the aged person a diet higher in proteins, vitamins, and minerals than would be theoretically necessary. The elderly are prone to suffer from protein deficiency more than from other forms of deficiency. Mild protein deficiency is made manifest by a sense of habitual fatigue. Severe protein deficiency results in loss of body tissue, damage to the organs of the body, impairment of body functions, and increased susceptibility to infections. Older persons also seem to lose some of the ability to absorb and use certain of the essential elements in food, especially calcium and iron. Calcium is needed to help prevent brittle and malformed bones, and iron is needed to combat the tendency toward anemia, especially in those persons who do not eat much meat. Many older persons do not eat enough meat because of the difficulty of chewing it. It is important that the meat be very tender or ground; stews and casseroles are good ways of serving it. Meat, fish, or poultry should be served at least once a day, and liver should be served once a week. The protein of meat should be supplemented by milk, eggs, and cheese. Milk and milk products are an excellent source of calcium and some of the necessary vitamins. Milk may also be given in the form of cream soups, other creamed dishes, and desserts. Dry milk may be added to a variety of foods. The adult need for vitamins remains the same as the years go by but may seem accentuated because the older person may be eating less food and generally utilizing it less well. Very often there is also reduced tolerance for fats. The diet should be plentifully supplied with milk, eggs, fruit, whole-grain products, and vegetables prepared in such a manner that the maximum content of the vitamins is retained. Sweets are used, but they should not replace the foods needed to furnish the body with the necessary proteins, vitamins, and minerals.

2. There should be sufficient calories for the maintenance of energy and activity. The caloric intake should be such as to avoid or correct underweight or obesity. The most desirable weight is the ideal weight at 25 years of age. If it is necessary for a patient to reduce, it should be done slowly and with a nutritionally sound diet plan. Sometimes aged persons eat to excess in order to alleviate boredom, loneliness, or anxiety. However, because metabolism slows down as they grow older, they do not need as many calories as formerly.

3. Diminshed secretion of mucus, which normally serves as a lubricant in the lower intestinal canal, contributes to the tendency toward constipation. Soft bulk is needed to prevent it. Cooked fruits and vegetables may be more easily chewed, swallowed, and digested than raw ones. Fruits stimulate the appetite as well as furnish bulk. Added fiber may be used also, along with adequate fluid intake.

4. Condiments and spices may be used according to individual taste, desire, or tolerance. Tasteless, bland food is neither appetizing nor satisfying and contributes to poor intake.

5. Meals consist of light, easily digested foods. A good breakfast should be the order of the day, and the evening meal should be substantial enough to prevent hunger during the night. A glass of milk or milk and crackers should be available in the evening if desired. Often, frequent small meals throughout the day meet needs better than regular meals.

6. Fluids are very important for the aged because a larger fluid intake, and therefore a larger urinary output, is needed to adequately eliminate the metabolic waste products. Sufficient fluids to produce at least 3 pints of urine a day are needed. This means a fluid intake of 2 quarts ordinarily and 3 quarts when the weather is very hot. Fluids can be taken as beverages, juices, and soups served at the meal. The kidneys must work harder to secrete a small amount of concentrated urine than a larger amount of dilute urine. Fluids are more readily absorbed and easier on the circulation if taken in small amounts at fairly frequent intervals, rather than in large amounts less frequently. Many older persons prefer most of the fluids to be hot.

7. Unless a patient is undernourished or senile, it is not advisable to coax him to eat more food that he wants. When the appetite is poor, especially if the will to live is weakened by long illness and helplessness, small, frequent feedings and easy-to-eat foods requiring very little effort to eat are best. Much of the food may be served in liquid form. Trays attractively served in an atmosphere of relaxation and at regular hours sometimes help to cheer a depressed patient and stimulate the appetite.

8. The likes and dislikes of the aged should be respected. When eating habits are poor, they can usually be improved if the change is made very gradually. New foods or different ways of cooking familiar foods must be introduced slowly.

Questions on nutrition

1. What are the advantages of breast-feeding?
2. At what age is the average breast-fed baby weaned?
3. What kinds of milk are used in artificial feeding?
4. Compare cow's milk with human milk.
5. What are the fluid requirements of a baby?
6. What are the protein needs of a baby?
7. How many calories per pound does a baby require?
8. Calculate the formula for an 8-pound baby 2 months of age.
9. Why does a baby require more calories per pound than an adult?
10. When is it usually necessary to give supplementary vitamin D?
11. In what way are the requirements different for a premature baby?
12. What is the best kind of milk for a premature baby and why?
13. Plan a diet for baby 4 months of age and one for a baby 8 months of age.
14. What are some of the problems in feeding a baby, and how can they be overcome?
15. What solid foods need to be added during the first year?

16. How does the growth pattern change in childhood years, and what is the result in the child's response to food?
17. How does good nutrition affect mental development?
18. What problems are involved in nutrition for an adolescent?
19. Why is it especially important for teenage girls to have a balanced diet?
20. What is responsible for the increase in life expectancy?
21. How does a well-balanced diet influence a person's years of usefulness?
22. What are three common nutritional errors among adults?
23. Even if reduction in food is necessary, what nutrients should always be supplied in adequate amounts?
24. How may sufficient protein be supplied in the diet?
25. What important changes in nutritional care during pregnancy have been recommended by the National Research Council?
26. What is an average gain in weight during pregnancy?
27. Why must the protein intake of a pregnant woman be increased?
28. What is the relationship of sufficient calories in the diet to the protein in the diet?
29. How may sufficient protein be supplied in the pregnant woman's diet?
30. Why are additional calcium, phosphorus, and vitamin D needed?
31. What other food factors need to be increased during pregnancy?
32. Why does a physician usually order a mineral-vitamin supplement during pregnancy?
33. What type of diet should be followed when vomiting is present during early pregnancy?
34. What are some of the causes of toxemia?
35. What type of diet is generally used in early stages of toxemia of pregnancy?
36. How many calories are in 1 ounce of human milk?
37. Why does an older person tend to have a protein deficiency?
38. Why does he need to receive a larger amount of protein, minerals, and vitamins than is theoretically necessary?
39. How may protein deficiency in an elderly person be avoided?
40. Why would it sometimes be necessary to give fat-soluble vitamins synthetically?
41. What is the best policy to use in reducing the weight of an obese older person?
42. Why does an older person sometimes have a tendency toward constipation, and how can this be prevented?
43. What is a reasonable guide for using seasonings in an older person's diet?
44. Why are fluids important?
45. Plan a 2-day diet for an older person.

Suggestions for additional study

1. Prepare a 2-day menu for an infant 8 months old.
2. Plan 2-day meals for each of the following: a 3-year-old child, a 6-year-old child, and an adolescent boy.
3. Make a complete study of the actual likes and dislikes of the average child 6 to 10 years of age.
4. Plan a diet for a pregnant woman.
5. Plan a diet for a nursing mother.
6. Visit an aged relative and discuss his eating habits. Chart his intake of food for 3 days and check it for adequacy.

References

Brewer, G. S.: What every pregnant woman should know. New York, 1977, Random House, Inc.

Brewer, T. H.: Metabolic toxemia of late pregnancy; a disease of malnutrition, Springfield, Ill., 1966, Charles C Thomas, Publisher.

Church, C. F., and Church, H. N.: Food values of portions commonly used, ed. 11, Philadelphia, 1970, J. B. Lippincott Co.

Committee on Maternal Nutrition, Food and Nutrition Board, National Research Council: Maternal nutrition and the course of pregnancy, Washington, D.C., 1970, National Academy of Sciences.

Food and Nutrition Board, National Academy of Sciences–National Research Council: Recommended dietary allowances, Washington, D.C., 1979, The Academy.

Primrose, T., and Higgins, A.: A study in human antepartum nutrition, J. Reprod. Med. 7:257, 1972.

Shank, R. E.: A chink in our armor, Nutrition Today 5(2):2, 1970.

Williams, S. R.: Nutrition and diet therapy, ed. 3, St. Louis, 1977, The C. V. Mosby Co., Chapters 17, 18, 20.

Williams, S. R.: Essentials of nutrition and diet therapy, ed. 2, St. Louis, 1978, The C. V. Mosby Co., Chapters 12-14.

Worthington, B. S., Vermeersch, J., and Williams, S. R.: Nutrition in pregnancy and lactation, St. Louis, 1977, The C. V. Mosby Co.

10

Planning menus for the family

The planning of a menu for a family is more complicated than planning for just one person because several different age groups are usually involved. However, the family menu should be planned in such a way that only a few variations are needed to adapt it to the various ages.

Menus should be planned to fit the family budget and to include all the foods needed to supply good nutrition. They should also have variety, and the food should be well prepared and attractively served. Menus may be planned according to The Basic Four Food Groups. A meal should have contrast in consistency as well as in color. For instance, a plate of creamed chicken, mashed potatoes, and creamed cauliflower would present no contrast in consistency or color. Even though it would be nutritious, it would be very unattractive.

Carefully planning the way in which a product is to be used is essential; a cheaper grade of canned vegetable or fruit may sometimes be used just as well as the more expensive ones. For example, tomatoes to be used in Swiss steak could just as well be Grade B. Cobblers or pies could be made from less expensive fruits canned especially for that purpose. The cheaper grades and the more expensive ones are essentially equal in value, and both grades are canned under equally sanitary conditions. Fresh fruits and vegetables may be used when they are in season.

Evaporated and dry skim milk are cheaper than fresh milk and are as good for cooking and many other purposes. Reconstituted dry skim milk is excellent for drinking if it is cold. Margarine is much cheaper than butter, and if it is fortified with vitamin A, it is equally nutritious.

The less expensive cuts of beef are as nutritious as expensive steaks. Pork or beef liver is much cheaper than calves' liver and is just as valuable a food. When the prices for meat are excessive, main dishes may be prepared from beans, peas, cheese, eggs, or peanut butter.

Generally, rolls, coffee cake, and cookies are cheaper if made at home than when purchased prepared. Cooked cereals such as oatmeal are cheaper than prepared cereals.

A nutritious breakfast is a good way to start the day. Family members may receive the recommended amount of vitamin C by serving orange juice, tomato juice, grapefruit, or grapefruit juice at this meal. A substantial breakfast consisting of orange juice, cereal with milk, and an egg will be more satisfying than a breakfast consisting of toast or sweet roll and coffee. Carbohydrates bring about a rapid rise in blood sugar and a subsequent rapid lowering of blood sugar, whereas proteins and fats, when eaten with the carbohydrates, will raise the blood sugar more slowly, resulting in a more lasting effect. A feeling of exhaustion is often the result of low blood sugar caused by eating a breakfast high in carbohydrate and low in protein and fat.

Dinner is the main meal of the day, whether it is served at night or in the middle of the day. For families in which some of the members eat the noon meal away from home, it is especially important that the protective foods be served at the evening meal.

Menus may be planned for a week in advance. Sometimes minor changes will be necessary, but the main framework of the menu can remain fairly constant. In planning the menus, place the protective foods (The Basic Four Food Groups) in the menu plan first and then add other foods to the menu as desired. (See Table 1-3, p. 9.)

The planning of menus in advance makes more economical buying possible and helps one to avoid the last-minute decision to prepare certain foods just because they can be prepared quickly. Processed, packaged, "convenience" foods are always more expensive than simple, bulk, primary foods.

MENUS FOR ONE WEEK FOR THE FAMILY

In the following menus, the foods that fulfill the requirements of The Basic Four Food Groups are printed in italics.

Breakfast	Lunch	Dinner
Monday		
Stewed prunes	Cream of tomato soup	*Roast beef*
Oatmeal	*Baked omelet*	Mashed potatoes
Crisp bacon	Chopped spinach	*Buttered peas*
Toast	*Celery sticks*	*Grapefruit and orange salad*
Butter or margarine	*Bread*	*Bread*
Milk	Butter or margarine	Butter or margarine
Coffee	Sugar cookies	Sponge cake with custard
	Milk for children	sauce
	Coffee for adults	*Milk*
		Coffee
Tuesday		
Orange juice	Cheese strata	*Baked pork chops*
Cream of Wheat	*Buttered string beans*	*Glazed sweet potatoes*
Soft-cooked egg	*Carrot sticks*	*Stewed tomatoes*

Breakfast	Lunch	Dinner
Toast	Butter or margarine	Lettuce salad
Butter or margarine	Fruit cup	*Bread*
Milk	*Milk* for children	Butter or margarine
Coffee	Coffee for adults	*Baked apple*
		Milk
		Coffee

Wednesday

Grapefruit sections	Vegetable soup	*Hamburger steaks*
Pettijohn's cereal	Old-fashioned hash	French fried potatoes
Poached egg	*Hot biscuits*	*Julienne carrots*
Toast	Sherbet	*Tomato salad*
Butter or margarine	*Milk* for children	*Bread*
Milk	Coffee for adults	Butter or margarine
Coffee		*Cherry cobbler*
		Milk
		Coffee

Thursday

Tomato juice	*Egg salad sandwich*	*Broiled liver*
Oatmeal	*Jellied fruit salad*	*Oven-browned potatoes*
Crisp bacon	Chocolate pudding	French fried onion rings
Toast	Applesauce cake	*Cabbage slaw*
Butter or margarine	*Milk* for children	*Bread*
Milk	Coffee for adults	Butter or margarine
Coffee		*Peach half*
		Milk
		Coffee

Friday

Orange juice	Cream of asparagus	*Baked haddock* with
Whole-wheat cereal	soup	tartar sauce
Scrambled eggs	Peanut butter and jelly	*Baked potato*
Toast	sandwich	*Harvard beets*
Butter or margarine	*Apricots*	*Celery hearts*
Milk	Oatmeal cookies	*Bread*
Coffee	*Milk* for children	Butter or margarine
	Coffee for adults	Lemon meringue pudding
		Milk
		Coffee

Saturday

Pineapple juice	Baked beans	*Veal stew* with potatoes
Cream of Wheat	*Tomato salad*	*Steamed cabbage*
with raisins	*Corn bread*	Pear and cottage cheese
Poached egg	Butter or margarine	salad
Toast	*Banana*	*Bread*
Butter or margarine	*Milk* for children	Butter or margarine
Milk	Coffee for adults	Gingerbread with orange
Coffee		sauce
		Milk
		Coffee

Breakfast	Lunch	Dinner
Sunday		
½ *grapefruit*	*Baked chicken* with	*Tuna salad sandwich*
Prepared cereal	dressing	*Pineapple* and American
Sausage links	*Mashed potatoes*	cheese salad
Toast	*Fresh broccoli*	Chocolate-covered
Butter or margarine	*Tossed salad*	graham crackers
Milk	*Bread*	*Milk*
Coffee	Butter or margarine	Coffee
	Ice cream	
	Milk for children	
	Coffee for adults	

Questions on planning menus for the family

1. What are some of the points to be considered in planning menus for a family?
2. What are some of the economy measures in planning a menu and in preparing the food?
3. Why is it beneficial to eat a nourishing breakfast?
4. Plan a well-balanced, nutritious breakfast.
5. Plan interesting menus for 3 days that will include the recommended daily allowances for good health, underlining the foods that are necessary to comply with The Basic Four requirements.

Suggestions for additional study

1. The students may be responsible for serving at one or more social functions so that they may gain a little insight into food service.
2. The students will benefit from field trips, such as touring a hospital kitchen, a meat-processing plant, or a dairy. This activity will broaden their outlook on the entire subject of food and its importance.

References

Williams, S. R.: Nutrition and diet therapy, ed. 3, St. Louis, 1977, The C. V. Mosby Co., Chapter 15.

Williams. S. R.: Essentials of nutrition and diet therapy, ed. 2, St. Louis 1978, The C. V. Mosby Co., Chapter 11.

11

Basic principles of cooking

MEATS, POULTRY, AND FISH

After meat, poultry, or fish is purchased, it should be unwrapped and covered loosely with waxed paper or foil and stored in the refrigerator. Ground meat that is not to be used the same day should be frozen. Freezing tenderizes meat somewhat; the lower the temperature the greater the tenderizing effect will be. Cured and smoked meats should not be frozen because their flavor deteriorates rapidly. Ham spoils more rapidly around the bone than elsewhere. However, ham can be safely refrigerated with the bone for 3 to 40 days, after which it is best to remove the meat from the bone and cover and store the meat in the refrigerator. The bone may be used for seasoning vegetables.

The methods used in cooking meat are divided into two general classifications: dry heat and moist heat. *Dry* heat, which is used for the more tender cuts of meat, consists of roasting, broiling, or panbroiling. Tender cuts include prime rib roasts, steaks or roasts from the loin and sirloin, leg of lamb, fresh pork loin, ham, lamb chops, and ground meat. *Moist* heat consists of braising, stewing, and simmering. The less tender cuts are the cuts used for pot roasts, Swiss steaks, braised meat casseroles, stews, and soups.

The different methods of cooking can be explained as follows:

Roast—to bake in an oven without added water, with or without covering
Broil—to cook by having direct heat over the meat
Panbroil—to cook uncovered in a frypan without the addition of any fat, turning frequently
Braise—to brown the meat in a little fat, add a small amount of liquid, and cook slowly
Stew—to brown small cubes of meat, add water to cover, and cook slowly
Simmer—to cook in a liquid at a temperature of 185° F.

Meats may be completely thawed or partially thawed before they are cooked. The cooking can be started when the meat is completely frozen, but the result in most cases is less satisfactory than when it is at least partially thawed. Thin pieces of meat may be cooked while they are still frozen, but thicker pieces of meat should be thawed before they are cooked. When meat is thawed in the refrigerator, there is less fluid drip than when it is thawed at room temperature. It takes about four to six times longer to thaw the meat in the refrigerator than it does to thaw it at room temperature.

Meats should be cooked at a low temperature, 300° to 325°F., except fresh pork, which should be cooked at 350° F. It is important that fresh pork be well done to eliminate the danger of trichinosis. Meat that is cooked at a low temperature is juicier, more tender, and more uniformly cooked, and it shrinks less. The brown color and the flavor desired in roasts are produced by long, slow cooking at a low temperature. Searing meat produces greater shrinkage and makes the meat drier.

A meat thermometer is very helpful, even to an experienced cook, since it is a more accurate means of determining the degree of "doneness" in a roast. The meat thermometer should be inserted through the thickest part of the roast at a place where it does not come in direct contact with the bone or with heavy layers of fat. The temperature of the oven and the internal temperature of various types of roasts when they are cooked are given in Table 11-1.

For broiling meat, the broiler should be rubbed with suet before each use. Broiling temperature is 350° F. If the oven temperature is 550° F. and the meat is placed 3 inches from the flame, the surface of the meat will be 350° F. The meat is placed 3 inches from the flame for a 2-inch steak and 2 inches for a 1-inch steak. The fat around the rim of the steak should be slashed to prevent curling. Pork should never be broiled because it requires more thorough cooking. Veal should not be broiled either. It responds best to long, slow cooking because of its low fat content and its large amount of connective tissue.

Poultry and fish should be thawed before they are cooked. Poultry should be washed thoroughly before it is used. Poultry is roasted by placing it on a rack in the roaster with the breast down. For the last half of the cooking time, the breast is turned up, and the bird can be basted with hot water and margarine (1 quart of hot water to 4 ounces of margarine). Do not cover the fowl or add water. If the chicken tends to brown too much toward the end of the roasting period, a piece of foil may be placed over the breast and drumsticks. The timetable for roasting chicken and turkey is given in Table 11-2.

Fish may be cooked at a little higher temperature (350° to 375° F.) for a short period of time. When the fish can be flaked with a fork, it is done. It should not be overcooked.

Table 11-3 lists the number of servings, oven temperature, and cooking time of various types of meat, poultry, and fish.

EGGS

Eggs should be refrigerated promptly. Eggs stored for 4 days at a temperature of 70° to 80° F. lose as much freshness as when they are stored in the re-

Table 11-1. Cooking temperatures for various types of roasts

Meat	Oven temperature (°F.)	Internal temperature as shown on meat thermometer (°F.)
Pork, fresh, well done	350	185
Ham, fresh, well done	350	185
Ham, cured, tenderized	325	160
Beef, roast, rare	325	140
Beef, roast, medium rare	325	160
Beef, roast, well done	325	170 to 175
Lamb, roast, well done	325	180
Veal, roast, well done	325	180

Table 11-2. Roasting time for chicken and turkey

Food item	Weight (lb.)	Temperature (°F.)	Approximate minutes per pound
Chicken, stuffed	4 to 5	325	35 to 40
Chicken, stuffed	5 to 7	325	20 to 25
Turkey, stuffed	8 to 10	325	20 to 25
Turkey, stuffed	10 to 16	325	18 to 20
Turkey, not stuffed	6	325	30
Turkey, not stuffed	8 to 10	325	20

Table 11-3. Number of servings, oven temperature, and cooking time for meats, poultry, and fish

Food item	Weight (lb.)	Approximate number of servings	Oven temperature (°F.)	Approximate minutes per pound
Prime ribs of beef	8	12	325	Rare, 18 to 20
Prime ribs of beef	8	12	325	Medium rare, 22 to 30
Prime ribs of beef	8	12	325	Well done, 30 to 40
Roast loin of pork	8	18	350	35 to 45
Roast leg of lamb	8	18	300	30 to 35
Roast veal leg	4	12	300	25 to 30
Baked ham, tenderized	12	20	325	20
Swiss steak	4	10	300	50
Meat loaf (beef and pork)	4	8 to 10	350	25
Baked chicken	5	6	350	20
Baked fish	3	6	325	Total of 25 to 30 min.

frigerator at 45° F. for several weeks. It is best to remove eggs from the refrigerator about 30 minutes beofre they are to be separated. Raw egg yolks
separate from the egg whites easier at 50° to 60° F. The white of an egg that is
just out of the refrigerator clings to both the shell and the yolk, making separa-
tion more difficult. Eggs should not be left out of the refrigerator longer than 30
minutes, because if the temperature of the egg reaches 75° F., the yolk is more
likely to break.

Hard-cooked eggs separate more easily from the shell if they are removed
promptly from the pan when they are cooked and placed in cold water. As soon
as the eggs are cool, they should be tapped gently as they are turned from side
to end, the shell being cracked in many places. They are then peeled under
cool running water, beginning at the large end of the egg.

Soiled eggs should not be washed until they are ready to be used. The
eggshell itself is porous, but it has a gelatinous coating that protects the inside
of the egg from germs or other contamination. Washing the egg removes this
protective coating and renders the contents of the egg more susceptible to contamination.

Eggs should be cooked at a low to moderate temperature. A high temperature and long cooking makes the egg white tougher and less digestible and
darkens the surface of the yolk. Any product that has eggs for the principal ingredient, such as custard, should be cooked at a low temperature.

Eggs perform many functions in the preparation of foods. They are a leaven-
ing agent; for example, beaten egg whites are added to cakes to make them
lighter. Eggs are emulsifiers, as in mayonnaise, in which they emulsify the oil
and vinegar. They are used as a thickening agent in custard and as a binding
agent in meat loaf. They act as adhesive agents; for example, croquettes are
dipped in eggs and then in crumbs. The egg clings to the croquette and holds
the crumbs, thus keeping the croquette in its original shape during frying. Eggs
are also a clarifying agent, as in coffee or soup.

Dried eggs are perishable after the can has been opened and must be refrigerated in a tightly covered container. Never reconstitute more than can be used
immediately. Dried eggs may be used in omelets, as scrambled eggs, and in
baked products. When they are used in a baked product, they can be mixed
with the dry ingredients, and the amount of water that would be used to recon-
situte the dried eggs is added to the amount of liquid used in the baked
product.

The following proportions may be used to reconstitute dried eggs:

$2^1/_2$ tbs. dried eggs and $2^1/_2$ tbs. water = 1 large egg
$^1/_3$ cup dried eggs and $^1/_3$ cup water = 2 large eggs
$^1/_2$ cup dried eggs and $^1/_2$ cup water = 3 large eggs

Because dried eggs tend to lump, it is necessary to sift them both before and
after they are measured to obtain a smooth product. After the second sifting,

the dried eggs should be sprinkled over the allowed amount of water and beaten until they are smooth.

DAIRY PRODUCTS
Milk

Milk should be promptly refrigerated. Most liquid milk is pasteurized. Pasteurization lessens the possibility of transmission of harmful bacteria and improves the keeping quality of the milk. Homogenized milk is milk in which the fat has been broken up into smaller globules. The fat globules are sufficiently reduced in size to prevent the formation of cream. Buttermilk, originally the by-product of butter, is now made in dairies. It is made from skimmed or partly skimmed milk by adding a culture of lactic acid bacilli. A portion of the milk sugar is changed to lactic acid by these harmless bacteria, and the milk has a softer, more finely divided curd.

Dry skim milk may be reconstituted or used in its dry form. Often it is reconstituted and mixed with fresh milk in proportions of one-half reconstituted dry skim milk and one-half fresh milk. The dry skim milk, either reconstituted or in the dry form, is excellent for baking and for any product in which milk is used. It may also be added in the dry form to whole milk when it is necessary or advisable to increase the protein in the diet or to increase the caloric content of the diet.

Milk should always be heated in a double boiler or at low heat because it scorches very easily, giving a very unpleasant taste to any product to which it is added.

Cheese

Cheese should not be frozen. When it is thawed, it becomes crumbly, and the flavor is changed. Processed cheese is not changed by freezing, but it will keep just as well in the refrigerator. Refrigeration stops natural aging of most cheeses. To obtain the best flavor, cheese should be removed from the refrigerator and allowed to reach room temperature before it is served. Cottage cheese is very perishable, and even with adequate refrigeration it should not be kept longer than 3 or 4 days.

Cheese or food containing cheese should always be cooked at a low temperature (325° F.). Cheese cooked at too high a temperature or for too long becomes stringy and rubbery, and the flavor and texture are definitely impaired. However, grated dry cheese used to top au gratin casseroles may be browned quickly at a higher temperature with no ill effects.

VEGETABLES

Most vegetables should be stored in a vegetable crisper or wrapped in cellophane and stored at 40° to 50° F. Potatoes should be stored in a cool place but not refrigerated. Vegetables must be washed thoroughly before they are used.

When vegetables are cooked, a minimum of water should be used, and they should not be overcooked. More vegetables are abused in cooking than any other groups of foods. Only the amount of the vegetable needed for one meal should be cooked. Vegetables that must be warmed over lose some of their vitamin and mineral content. Frozen vegetables need not be thawed before they are cooked but should be broken apart so that they will cook uniformly throughout.

Fresh spinach and other greens need have no water added since enough water clings to the leaves to prevent burning.

If fresh asparagus is prepared, the bottom of the stems should be removed at the point where they break easily, and the scales should be removed from the stalk that is to be cooked. Asparagus stalks should be tied together and cooked with the heads up so that they will be cooked by the steam and will not be overcooked. If cut asparagus is prepared, the tips should not be added until after the stems have cooked for 10 minutes.

The damaged outside leaves should be removed from lettuce, and the core should be cut out. A head of lettuce should be held under cold running water until the leaves become loosened and can be separated and drained. The leaves may then be refrigerated for a few hours to finish the crisping.

Cauliflower may be cooked as a whole head, or the flowerets may be separated from the core before it is cooked.

Tomatoes that are to be peeled should be dipped in boiling water for a few seconds until the skins become loosened. They are then refrigerated, and the skins are removed just before the tomatoes are used.

Beets are washed and cooked, and the skins are removed. About an inch of the stems should remain on beets while they are cooking to prevent them from bleeding. Onions can be peeled under water to prevent discomfort for the worker.

If any water remains in the kettle after vegetables have been cooked, it should be saved and used in soups. Any excess liquid from canned peas, string beans, lima beans, or corn should also be saved and used in soups.

Strong-flavored vegetables should be cooked uncovered so that the volatile substances are released. Otherwise, these substances will react on the sulfur content of the vegetables and produce compounds that are not only disagreeable in odor and flavor but that are also difficult to digest. The strong-flavored vegetables are broccoli, Brussels sprouts, cauliflower, cabbage, and onions. All other vegetables should be covered while they are cooking.

MISCELLANEOUS FOODS
Fruits

Most fruits, except bananas, should be stored at 40° to 50° F. Bananas should be stored at room temperature, or 70° F. Frozen fruits should be stored in the freezer until they are ready to be used.

Fruit that is to be used for a pie or a cobbler should be thawed in the container in which it came. The juice should be drained off and thickened with cornstarch, cooked, and then poured back over the fruit and allowed to cool before the fruit is used. The following amounts of frozen fruits are used for pies:

4 cups prepared fruit for 9-inch pie
$2^2/_3$ cups prepared fruit for 8-inch pie
$2^1/_4$ cups prepared fruit for 7-inch pie
$1^2/_3$ cups prepared fruit for 6-inch pie

Frozen fruits make delicious desserts. When the fruit is placed in the serving dishes, it should be just partially thawed or even have a few small ice crystals.

Salads

For salads, the ingredients must be chilled, and the lettuce must be crisp and cold. Dressings must be added at the last minute unless they are a part of the salad, as in chicken salad or potato salad. Vegetable and fruit salads are best if all the ingredients are prepared in advance, stored separately, and then assembled at the last minute.

Molded salads should be made with care. All the gelatin must be dissolved, and the gelatin mixture should be partially congealed before well-drained fruit or vegetables are added. The salad is unmolded by careful insertion of a silver knife around the edge of the mold no deeper than 1 inch. The pan is then held in hot water for a second or two, and the salad is gently separated from the mold.

Sandwiches

Thin tea sandwiches are made from unsliced bread, which is placed in a refrigerator for 2 hours to make it more firm. It is then sliced in thin slices. Crusts are not trimmed off until after the sandwiches are made. If the sandwiches are not to be used immediately, they should be covered well with waxed paper or foil.

Frozen foods

Once frozen foods have been thawed, they must not be refrozen. Not only is the quality of the product impaired, but there is also danger of contamination. If the entire amount of the frozen product cannot be used, the package should be divided with a sharp knife or a small saw made for this purpose, and the unused portion should be returned to the freezing compartment.

Questions on basic principles of cooking

1. How should meat be stored?
2. Why should ham not be frozen?
3. Where does ham spoil the quickest?
4. What are the two general methods of cooking meat?
5. What specific methods are included in each of the two methods? Explain each.

6. Should meat be thawed before cooking? Discuss.
7. What temperatures should be used for cooking meats?
8. Why should meat be cooked at a low temperature?
9. Of what advantage is a meat thermometer?
10. How should it be inserted?
11. How should meat be broiled?
12. Why should pork and veal not be broiled?
13. How should poultry be roasted?
14. How does one determine when fish is cooked?
15. Why should eggs be taken out of the refrigerator before the time that they are to be used?
16. What is the best way to remove shells from hard-cooked eggs?
17. Why should soiled eggs not be washed?
18. Why should a low temperature be used for cooking eggs?
19. List at least four functions of eggs in the preparation of other foods.
20. How are dried eggs reconstituted?
21. Why is milk pasteurized?
22. How does homogenized milk differ from milk that has not been homogenized?
23. How is buttermilk made?
24. What are some of the uses of dry skim milk?
25. How should milk be heated and why?
26. How should cheeses be stored?
27. Why should a low temperature be used for cooking cheese or foods containing cheese?
28. Name one exception in which cheese may be subjected to a higher temperature.
29. Give some of the principles for cooking vegetables.
30. What use should be made of liquids left over from canned vegetables?
31. Which vegetables should be covered during cooking and which vegetables should not be covered? Why?
32. Which fruit should not be refrigerated?
33. Discuss the use of frozen fruit.
34. Discuss the proper procedure in making salads. Discuss the procedure for making sandwiches.
35. Why should frozen foods not be refrozen after they have been thawed?

Suggestions for additional study

1. Cook one 4-pound beef rib roast at 325° F. and another 4-pound beef rib roast at 450° F. Compare the two finished products as to cooked weight, degree of juiciness, and flavor.
2. Freeze a small piece of cheese and note the results after it has thawed.
3. Boil an egg for 30 to 40 minutes and observe the dark rim around the yolk.

References

American Heart Association: The American Heart Association Cookbook, New York, 1973, David McKay Co., Inc.

Gates, J. C.: Basic foods, New York, 1976, Holt, Rinehart and Winston.

Jones, J.: Diet for a happy heart, San Francisco, 1975, 101 Productions.

Jones, J.: Fabulous fiber cookbook, San Francisco, 1977, 101 Productions.

Jones, J.: The calculating cook: a gourmet cookbook for diabetics and dieters, San Francisco, 1972, 101 Productions.

12

The community food supply and its relation to health

The health of any community is directly dependent on the food supply available to its people and their personal choices from that supply. Thus, the community food environment and individual food habits of persons living in that environment become primary concerns basic to all well-being and happiness.

Over the past few years the American food environment has been rapidly changing. Knowledge of food science and technology has greatly expanded. As a result, the number of processed foods in modern supermarkets, as well as the number of "fast food" chains, has increased markedly, replacing many primary food items in the diets of many people. These changes bring both promise and problems the promise of abundance and variety in the food supply and problems of increasing confusion in food identity and values, with increasing consumption of food additives and nonnutritive products.

To safeguard the community food supply, every detail of food production must always be carefully watched to protect the nutrients, to prevent contamination from harmful bacteria and other organisms, and to eliminate toxic substances. A safe water supply has been ensured in most communities. Milk and dairy products are produced under sanitary conditions. Infected cows have been eliminated, and raw milk is pasteurized for most of our population. It now remains for other items of food to be made equally safe.

The history of public concern over the safety of its food supply goes back to 1906, when the first Pure Food and Drug Act was passed. However, not much was done until 1938, when our present law, the Federal Food, Drug, and Cosmetic Act, came into existence and created the Food and Drug Administration (FDA). The FDA, operating under the Department of Health, Education, and Welfare (HEW), is now the federal agency that is charged with the responsibility of protecting the public from contaminated or inferior products, inaccurate labeling, and harmful additives.

It was not until 1958 that increasing consumer concern caused Congress to pass the first amendment to this basic food safety law. This regulation, the Food Additives Amendment, was passed in September 1958 and became fully effective in March 1959 for all new chemical additives. The law provided for the first time that no additive could be used in food unless the FDA, after a careful review of the testing results, agreed that the compound was safe at the intended levels of usage. The amendment made an exception for all additives in use at that time that were "generally recognized as safe" (GRAS). In addition, in the final hours of debate on the bill, Congress added the Delaney clause, which states that no additive that is found to induce cancer in humans or animals by ingestion or testing shall be allowed as safe. It was under this clause that cyclamates were banned in 1969.

The result of the Food Additives Amendment of 1958-1959 has been the establishment of what is now know as the GRAS list. This list contains a large number of food additives that are "generally recognized as safe" but have not undergone rigid testing requirements. Problems, however, exist with this GRAS list. The number of food additives on the list is uncertain. and the use of them has greatly increased as the number of processed foods has increased. As a result, the federal government has now directed the FDA to reevaluate all the items on the GRAS list for safety. Food additives in general are facing increasing public awareness and concern.

This increasing consumer concern about food products has brought about changes in regulations controlling food labels. In 1967 regulations were adopted that required more complete and more prominent information on the labels of packaged foods. These "truth in packaging" laws sought to regulate "special diet" foods, especially vitamin and mineral supplements and so-called low-calorie foods. Then in 1973 came the new nutrient-labeling regulations that were mandatory throughout the food industry by the end of 1974. In essence, these laws regulate dietary supplementation by requiring that any food product making a nutrient claim must support that claim with specific nutrient information on the label. Market competition will no doubt extend the practice of including nutrient information on the labels of an increasing number of food products. Nutritional labeling is here to stay. A "nutrition revolution" has begun. Once people begin to understand the relationship between sound nutrition and good health, they will demand nutritional labeling and education, just as they demand a responsible environmental policy to control pollution.

FOOD-BORNE DISEASES AND CHEMICAL POISONING

After canned foods, meat, milk, and other food products have been produced under the most favorable conditions and their processing and marketing have been controlled by the government regulations, there are still many possibilities of contamination with disease-producing organisms by careless food handlers. Unnecessary human contact with food should be avoided, and periodic health examinations should be required of all food handlers.

Frequent washing of the hands by food handlers is *essential*. Correct dish-washing is another important phase of food sanitation. Dishes and silverware should be allowed to drain dry. Constant attention to cleanliness and sanitation is important to health.

Various food-borne diseases result from eating contaminated food or from harmful chemicals in food.

1. Bacterial contamination of food by the organisms causing tuberculosis, the common cold, dysentery, typhoid, and septic sore throat has become a serious health problem. The source of trouble is usually food improperly refrigerated or prepared under unsanitary conditions. These organisms multiply rapidly in semisoft foods, which allows them to go through the entire mass quickly. Custard pie, cream puffs, and ground-meat mixtures are rich environments for the growth of these organisms. Another frequent way in which harmful organisms are passed around is by food handlers who may be carriers of one or more diseases.

2. Food poisoning may result from eating fruits and vegetables treated with chemicals, especially lead and arsenic. All fruits and vegetables should be washed very thoroughly before they are used.

3. Botulism is the most serious form of food poisoning. It usually occurs when home-canned foods have been underprocessed. The toxin can grown only in containers from which air is excluded, such as sealed cans. The foods in which it most often occurs are meats, fish, and vegetables low in acid, such as asparagus, beans, beets, and corn. The toxin is absorbed directly from the digestive tract, and within 12 to 24 hours it acts on the nervous system, causing abdominal cramps, double vision, and difficulty in swallowing. Later, nausea, vomiting, and diarrhea develop. It proves fatal in approximately 65% of patients within 3 to 7 days.

4. Certain diseases can be transmitted from animals to humans. Trichinosis results from eating raw or improperly cooked pork from an animal that was infested with the trichina organism. Tularemia may be transmitted to humans from infected rodents, especially rabbits. Undulant fever may be contracted from drinking the milk of an infected cow.

5. Mushrooms that have not been grown commercially should never be used, since certain varieties growing in the wild state are poisonous.

6. DDT and other insecticides used as surface sprays can be harmful. It is estimated that a teaspoon of DDT would be fatal. However, even more poisonous to humans is sodium fluoride powder. Neither substance should be used around food-preparation areas, except with extreme caution. In fact, all the newer insecticides must be used with caution around food and food-preparation areas. This applies to all powders, vapors, dusts, and liquid preparations. No product should be used unless the active chemical ingredient is declared on the label. Poisonous liquids or powders should never be stored in an unlabeled container or even in the same storage area as food.

Questions on food and its relation to health

1. When was the first Food and Drug Act passed?
2. What is the significance of the Food Additives Amendment that was passed in September 1958 and the subsequent GRAS list?
3. What is the role of the FDA in relationship to the food supply?
4. What are the nutrient labeling regulations?
5. Name three points that would be considered important for the sanitary handling of food.
6. What are some of the possible causes of bacterial contamination of food?
7. What is the common cause of botulism?
8. Name some diseases that may be transmitted from animals to humans.
9. What precautions should be taken in using insecticides?

Suggestions for additional study

1. If you are in a hospital, ask the laboratory to prepare a slide showing the germs on dishes that have been improperly washed or on clean dishes that have been handled by unclean hands.
2. Secure a film from your city health department on any of the phases of sanitation.
3. Visit a local food market and make a survey of food labels. What information do you find on them?

References

Johnson, O. C.: The Food and Drug Administration and labeling, J. Am. Diet. Assoc. **64:**471, 1974.

Protecting our food: Yearbook of Agriculture, 1966, Washington, D.C., 1966, U. S. Government Printing Office.

Ross, M. L.: What's happening to food labeling? J. Am. Diet. Assoc. **64:**263, 1974.

Williams, S. R.: Nutrition and diet therapy, ed. 3, St. Louis, 1977, The C. V. Mosby Co., Chapter 12.

Williams, S. R.: Essentials of nutrition and diet therapy, ed. 2, St. Louis, 1978, The C. V. Mosby Co., Chapter 9.

13

Food habits and nationality food patterns

Food habits do not develop in a vacuum. They are formed from birth throughout life as a response to many influences, which include a person's culture and family, his social class and setting, his economic situation, and multiple psychological and emotional factors. These food habits are deeply rooted and become the basis of personal food choices. Food has many meanings, and a person's food habits are intimately tied up with his whole way of life. It is important in the health care of any person to recognize this basic fact in food behavior.

A number of nationality or cultural group food patterns are represented in American community life. Several of these are briefly listed here. Note unusual traditional foods in each group.

ITALY

The Italian foods include goat's milk, cheese, eggs, macaroni, dark breads, olive oil, garlic, green peppers, wine and other liquors, soup made from meat stock and vegetables, and polenta. The Italian diet, especially for children, could include more milk, coarse cereals, root vegetables, and potatoes and less candy and coffee.

HUNGARY

The Hungarian foods include the grains, potatoes, fresh and cured pork, highly seasoned foods, paprika, onions, and green and red fresh peppers. The diet also includes sour cream, sauerkraut, fish, shrimp, eggs, and fruits. The Hungarians could include more raw vegetables, cereals, and milk in their diet.

POLAND

The Polish foods include potatoes, rye bread, buckwheat flour, coarse cereals cooked in milk, pork (especially highly seasoned sausage), fresh, salted, or pickled fish, cabbage (raw, cooked, and as sauerkraut), vegetables cooked with meat, sour cream, and cottage cheese. More milk, raw vegetables, and fruit could be included in the Polish people's diet.

TURKEY AND GREECE

The foods most characteristic of diets in Turkey and Greece are fruits, vegetables, meats rich in fat (lamb is the favorite), gravies, and yoghurt, a sour milk preparation.

MEXICO

The Mexican foods include the many varieties of beans, rice, potatoes, tomatoes, and some other vegetables, chili pepper, chili con carne, meat that is freshly slaughtered, tamales, and tortillas. The Mexican diet could contain more milk for children and more cheese and whole-grain breads.

PORTUGAL

The foods that are most charactreistic of Portugal, together with their meats, vegetables, and fruits, are grains other than wheat, spices (especially allspice and mace), and peppers.

CHINA

The characteristic foods in the Chinese diet are fermented eggs (hen, duck, and pigeon), cereals, vegetables, sprouts such as bean and bamboo, soybeans, rice, millet cakes in north China, noodles, sweet potatoes, some pork, lamb, and beef (must be chopped because of an ancient law of Confucius), some buffalo milk, coagulated blood, and fish and shellfish, which are sold alive. The chief food lacking in the Chinese diet is milk.

PUERTO RICO

The foods that are most widely used in Puerto Rico are rice, beans, salted codfish, pork, sweet potatoes and other root vegetables, bananas, and oranges. The chief food lacking in the diet of the Puerto Rican people is milk.

JAPAN

The principal foods in the Japanese diet are large amounts of cereals, potatoes and other vegetables, and seafood. More milk could be used.

LEBANON

Food to an Arab is an important item. Most of the Arab dishes take hours of preparation and are mixtures of various foods. The most characteristic foods of the Lebanese are Arabic coffee in the early morning, hot boiled milk at breakfast (boiled because of the prevalence of bacteria), cheese, olives, leban, which is made from whole milk and yeast (lebni is leban with the whey removed), eggs, butter and bread, meats (preferably mutton), Semnah (a heavy mutton fat), Mashi, which is vegetables with meat and rice, and milk pudding.

THE JEWISH PEOPLE

The principal meats used in the Jewish people's diet are cattle, sheep, goat, deer, and antelope (animals that have the cloven hoof and chew their cud). Other foods include haddock, halibut, salmon, tuna, pike, trout, buffalo, carp, whitefish, and perch (fish that have scales and fins), borscht, vegetable soup, Passover cake with potato flour, and matzo balls.

For Passover the symbols of Passover are placed at the head of the table. These symbolic food items are three matzoth, bitter herbs, a lamb bone, and haroses, a dish made of apples, nuts, cinnamon, and wine mixed together.

Other foods in the Jewish people's diet are tomato soup, wine soup, sauerkraut soup, mixed fruit soup, gefilte fish, baked broilers, beef pot roast, roast beef with vegetables, meat and carrot tzimmes, beef with prunes and sweet potatoes, carrot sticks in honey, potato kugel, kosher dill pickles, blintzes, kreplach dough, schnecken, and strudel.

Questions on foods used by various countries
1. How are food habits formed?
2. Name at least three foods used in each of the cultural groups discussed in the chapter.

References
Williams, S. R.: Nutrition and diet therapy, ed. 3, St. Louis, 1977, The C. V. Mosby Co., Chapter 13.

Williams, S. R.: Essentials of nutrition and diet therapy, ed. 2, St. Louis, 1978, The C. V. Mosby Co., Chapter 10.

PART THREE

DIET THERAPY

14

Routine hospital diets

The dietary treatment of the sick is a threefold responsibility that rests upon the physician, the dietitian or clinical nutrition specialist, and the nurse. Only by perfect teamwork can the best results be obtained.

The beginnings of dietary service to hospital patients can be traced to Florence Nightingale's work during the Crimean War in 1854. She did much to improve food service as well as nursing care. The nursing profession was, for many years, responsible for the dietary work in hospitals. The first resident teacher of sickroom cookery, a graduate of an Eastern cooking school, was employed at Johns Hopkins Hospital in 1890 to instruct the nurses in cooking. Other hospitals followed this example. At first this cooking teacher was called "superintendent of diet" and later "dietitian." Today the modern dietitian is an applied food scientist skilled in meeting the nutritional needs of people in a variety of settings and situations.

Nutrition, in comparison with medicine and nursing, is an infant science. Most of the information about nutrition in relation to treatment of disease has been learned in the last 40 years.

We all know that good food is essential to health. This is an accepted fact, but seldom do people realize how often poor selection of food is a contributory factor in disease.

Nutrition has become a very important subject to the nursing, dietary, and medical professions. The wide interest in foods and the ready acceptance of food fads make it all the more necessary that the dietitian, nurse, and physician take every opportunity to give correct dietary information to the public.

The normal well-balanced diet is the basis for all dietary prescriptions. The therapeutic diet should be adequate if at all possible. It should be evaluated, and if any nutrient is not present in sufficient quantity, supplements should be given. If, for instance, a patient is allergic to all milk products, then certain vitamin concentrates as well as calcium supplements may be necessary.

The objects of dietary treatment are as follows:
1. To increase or decrease weight

2. To allow a particular organ of the body to rest, as in the restriction of fat in diseases of the gallbladder
3. To plan the diet to correspond with the body's ability to metabolize a certain nutrient, as in diabetes
4. To remedy conditions due to deficiencies, such as the deficency of vitamin D in rickets
5. To eliminate certain harmful substances from the diet, such as caffeine, alcohol, and pepper in peptic ulcer disease

Modifications of the normal diet may be made as necessary to meet the needs of the patient in relation to the disease. Calories may be decreased or increased. Modifications may be made in the balance of nutrients, such as high or low protein, carbohydrate, fat, minerals, or vitamins. Certain foods may be omitted, as in cases of allergy.

Modifications in consistency are made in the following routine hospital diets: regular, soft, mechanical soft, medical liquid, and surgical liquid.

The regular diet is almost unlimited in the foods that may be served. The soft diet contains only very tender meats and tender cooked vegetables, such as carrots, asparagus, and beets. Vegetables containing much fiber should be omitted or pureed. Peaches, pears, applesauce, Royal Anne cherries, and grapefruit and orange sections that are free of membrane may be served on this diet. Coarse breads and cereals are omitted, as are highly spiced foods. Plain cake, puddings, and desserts are allowed.

The mechanical soft diet is a modification of the soft diet, in that all foods must be very soft or ground. The mechanical soft diet is used when for various reasons a patient cannot chew or use the facial muscles.

The medical, or full, liquid diet includes any food that is liquid at body temperature. Thin, strained cereal gruel is also served on this diet. Foods in the liquid state are easier to digest because they are so finely divided. Feedings should be given six times a day on liquid diets.

The surgical, or clear, liquid diet includes clear broth, tea, black coffee, and flavored gelatin.

Routine hospital diets are summarized in Table 14-1.

The patient's tray should be attractively arranged with colorful foods. The dishes, glasses, and utensils should be gleaming, the tray cover and napkins should be immaculate, and each item should be placed on the tray in an orderly manner. Arrangement of standard items should be the same at each meal. The tray should be large enough so that it does not look crowded. The use of chipped or cracked dishes or mixed patterns should be avoided. Servings should not be too large, because large servings are not so attractive as smaller portions, and they tend to discourage a patient, especially if he has little desire to eat. In order to appeal to the patient, hot foods must be served hot and cold foods cold. Hot foods, as well as salads and desserts, should be arranged attrac-

Table 14-1. Routine hospital diets

	Clear liquid	Full liquid	Soft	Light	Regular
Soup	Broth, bouillon	Same, plus strained soups	Same	All	All
Cereal		Thin cereal gruel	Refined cooked cereals, cornflakes, rice, noodles, macaroni, spaghetti	Same	All
Bread			White bread, crackers, melba toast, zwieback	Same, plus graham and rye bread	All
Protein foods		Milk, cream, milk drinks	Same, plus eggs (not fried), mild cheese, fowl, fish, sweetbreads, tender beef, veal, lamb, liver, bacon, gravy	Same	All
Vegetables			Potatoes: baked, mashed, creamed, steamed, escalloped; tender cooked whole bland vegetables (may be strained or puréed)	Same, cooked whole bland	All
Fruit and fruit juices	Apple juice	All	Same, plus bland cooked fruit: peaches, pears, applesauce, peeled apricots, white cherries, banana, orange and grapefruit sections without membrane		
Desserts and gelatin	Plain gelatin, water ice	Same, plus sherbet, ice cream, puddings, custard	Same, plus plain sponge cakes, plain cookies, plain cake, simple puddings	Same	All
Miscellaneous	Ginger ale, carbonated water, coffee, tea	Same	Same, plus butter, salt, pepper	Same	

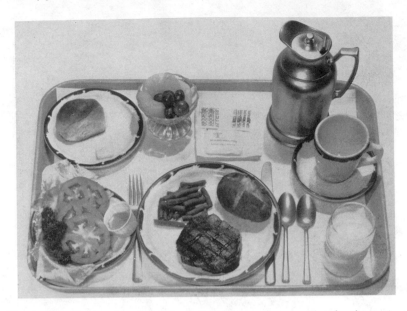

Fig. 2 Tray arrangement that is both attractive and convenient for the patient.

tively on the plate. Color combinations should be considered. The person who serves the tray should be sure that everything is within reach of the patient and that everything about the tray is correct before he leaves the patient. Nothing is more exasperating to a patient, for example, than to receive a pot of hot water and no tea bag.

Fig. 2 shows a tray arrangement that is neat as well as in logical order for the patient's convenience.

Each patient must be treated as an individual. It should be remembered that hospitalized patients are sick persons and may not be their normal selves. They may not want to eat. Their appetites should be tempted if possible, and they should be sympathetically treated at all times. The person who takes the tray to the patient should do so with a smile and a pleasant word. If the patient must be fed, the nurse should be very patient and not try to feed too rapidly. It is not necessary or desirable to keep up a rapid conversation, but if the patient is well enough to be interested, a little pleasant conversation will add pleasure in the meal. When a patient is happy with his food, both the physician and the nurse find treatment easier.

Questions on routine hospital diets

1. What were some of the beginnings of dietetics?
2. What is the basis of a therapeutic diet?
3. What are the objects of dietary treatment?
4. In what ways may the regular diet be modified?
5. Plan a soft diet for a patient who is allergic to milk products.
6. Plan a high-calorie medical liquid diet.

Suggestion for additional study

1. Interview the administrative dietitian or food service manager in your community hospital and observe the mode of patient food service. Report your findings to your class.

References

Williams, S. R.: Nutrition and diet therapy, ed. 3, St. Louis, 1977, The C. V. Mosby Co., Chapter 23.

Williams, S. R.: Essentials of nutrition and diet therapy, ed. 2, St. Louis, 1978, The C. V. Mosby Co., Chapter 15.

15

Modifications in individual constituents

The dietary changes discussed in this chapter are modifications of a regular well-balanced diet. Since it would be impractical to describe a diet each time it is discussed in subsequent chapters, the most commonly used diets are described in detail in this chapter.

HIGH-CALORIE DIET (APPROXIMATELY 4,000 CALORIES)

In a high-calorie diet emphasis is placed on increasing the calories rather than on increasing any particular nutrient. A full meal should be eaten three times a day, with a substantial snack in the afternoon and in the evening. This fifth meal may consist of a sandwich and milk shake or whatever else the person may wish.

This diet is adequate in all nutrients. The following foods should be included in the daily diet (other foods may be eaten as desired):

Beverages	4 cups milk, 1 large glass fruit juice
Bread	6 slices, whole-wheat or enriched
Butter or margarine	2 tbs. or more
Cereal	1 large serving, whole-wheat or enriched
Cheese	As desired
Cream	$1/2$ cup at breakfast
Desserts	Pie, cake, ice cream, or cookies as desired
Eggs	1 daily
Fruit	1 serving fruit in addition to large glass fruit juice at breakfast
Meat, fish, or poultry	2 large servings
Potato or potato substitutes	2 servings daily
Vegetables	At least 3 vegetables (1 raw and 1 green or yellow)
Soups	As desired

SAMPLE MENU

Breakfast	Lunch	Dinner
1 large glass orange juice	3¹/₂ oz. portion leg of lamb	1 medium club steak,
³/₄ cup oatmeal	³/₄ cup mashed potatoes	broiled
¹/₂ cup light cream	¹/₂ cup peas and carrots with	Large baked potato with
1 soft-cooked egg with	with butter	butter or margarine
butter or margarine	Pineapple and cream cheese	Spinach with vinegar
3 tsp. sugar	salad	Tomato salad with 1 tbs.
2 strips bacon	Hot biscuit	French dressing
1 slice toast	1 tsp. butter or margarine	1 slice bread
1 tsp. butter or margarine	Lemon meringue pie	1 tsp. butter or margarine
1 cup milk	1 cup milk	Baked apple with cream
Coffee if desired		1 glass milk
	3 P.M.	**8 P.M.**
	¹/₂ cup ice cream	Chocolate malted milk
	2 sugar cookies	
	1 glass milk	

HIGH-PROTEIN DIET (APPROXIMATELY 100 GRAMS)

A high-protein diet is a normal diet with added amounts of meat, milk, eggs, cheese, fish, or poultry. Nonfat dry milk may be added to soups or to regular milk, thereby increasing the protein without increasing the fat. A protein supplement may also be used. This diet is adequate in all nutrients. The daily diet should include the following foods:

Beverages	3 glasses milk
Cereals	1 whole-grain or enriched
Cheese	May be used freely
Eggs	3 eggs (1 or 2 may be used in cooking)
Fruit	At least 2 servings (1 a citrus fruit or fruit juice)
Meat, fish, or poultry	2 large servings each day
Potatoes or potato	1 serving daily
substitutes	
Vegetables	3 servings (1 raw and 1 green or yellow)
Bread, butter or margarine,	As desired
desserts, and soups	

SAMPLE MENU

Breakfast	Lunch	Dinner
¹/₂ grapefruit	4 oz. roast beef	Beef and vegetable soup
2 eggs	Mashed potatoes	2 lamb chops
2 slices crisp bacon	Buttered peas	Buttered asparagus
Toast	Combination vegetable salad	Peach and cottage cheese
Butter or margarine	Whole-wheat bread	salad
Coffee with cream	Butter or margarine	Whole-wheat bread
Milk	Fruit cup	Butter or margarine
	Milk	Baked custard
		Milk

LOW-PROTEIN DIET (APPROXIMATELY 40 GRAMS)

This diet contains only about 40 grams of protein and is usually given for only a short time. One ounce only of meat, poultry, fish, or cheese is allowed daily. One cup of milk and one egg may be taken daily.

Three slices of bread may be eaten daily. Cereals with cream and sugar may be served at breakfast. All fruits may be used, as well as all vegetables except dried peas and beans. Butter may be used as desired.

Broth soups and cream soups made with part of the milk allowance may be taken. Simple puddings may be made from the milk allowance.

A low-protein diet is inadequate in protein, calcium, iron, and all of the vitamins except ascorbic acid.

SAMPLE MENU

Breakfast	Lunch	Dinner
½ grapefruit	1 cup potato soup	1 oz. roast beef
1 egg	Fruit plate	Baked potato with butter or
Cereal with cream	Jelly sandwich	margarine
Toast	Sherbet	Fresh asparagus
Butter or margarine	Tea	Buttered carrots
Strawberry preserves		Tomato salad
Coffee with cream		Applesauce
		Coffee with cream

HIGH-CARBOHYDRATE DIET

The high-carbohydrate diet should include the following foods in the daily diet.

Beverages	Fruit juice as desired, 1 qt. milk
Bread	2 slices at each meal
Cereals	1 large serving whole-grain or enriched
Desserts	Cake, cookies, ice cream, sherbet, pastries that are not too rich, and puddings
Eggs	1 daily
Meat, fish, or poultry	2 servings
Fruits	2 servings (1 a citrus fruit or fruit juice)
Potato or potato substitute	2 servings
Vegetables	3 servings (1 raw and 1 green or yellow)
Butter, cheese, and soups	As desired

SAMPLE MENU

Breakfast	Lunch	Dinner
Orange juice	Fruit juice cocktail	Broiled chicken
Stewed prunes	Creamed chipped beef on	Candied sweet potatoes
Oatmeal with cream	toast	Buttered peas
Scrambled eggs	Baked potato with butter or	Pineapple and banana salad
2 slices toast	margarine	2 slices whole-wheat bread
Butter or margarine	Glazed carrots	Butter or margarine
Jelly	Apple and celery salad	Caramel cake
Coffee	Sherbet	Milk
Milk	Milk	

LOW-FAT DIET

A low-fat diet is a normal diet with increased amounts of carbohydrate and protein and a limited amount of fat.

No fried foods are used. Meats are broiled, boiled, or baked, without the additon of any fat. All visible fat is removed from the cooked meat. No pork or other meat high in fat content should be eaten. All foods are cooked without the addition of any fat. One egg and 3 teaspoons of butter are allowed per day. Skimmed milk is used in place of whole milk, Ice cream is not permitted, but sherbet is allowed. This diet is inadequate in the fat-soluble vitamins. The daily diet should include the following foods:

Beverages	Skimmed milk or buttermilk made from skimmed milk
Butter or margarine	3 tsp. only
Cheese	Cottage cheese only
Desserts	Gelatin, sherbet, and fruit desserts
Eggs	One daily, prepared without fat
Fruits	As desired (1 citrus)
Meat, fish, or poultry	Lean (may be roasted, broiled, or boiled)
Soups	Broths free from fat or soup made with skimmed milk
Bread, cereals, potato, potato substitutes, and other vegetables	As desired

SAMPLE MENU

Breakfast	Lunch	Dinner
Orange juice	Beef broth	Lean roast beef
Wheat cereal	Sliced white meat of chicken	Parsley potatoes
Poached egg	Baked potato with 1 tsp.	Sliced carrots
Toast	butter or margarine	Shredded lettuce salad
1 tsp. butter or margarine	Green beans	Whole-wheat bread
Coffee	Tomato salad	1 tsp. butter or margarine
Skimmed milk	Whole-wheat bread	Gelatin with fruit
	Jelly	Skimmed milk or tea
	Canned peach halves	
	Skimmed milk	

MINIMUM-FAT DIET

In the minimum fat diet the same restrictions are necessary as for the low fat diet, except that no egg or butter is allowed.

Since this diet is often given to patients with disorders of the gallbladder, raw vegetables and all raw fruits except citrus fruits are omitted from the diet.

This diet is inadequate in the fat-soluble vitamins.

SAMPLE MENU

Breakfast	Lunch	Dinner
Orange juice	Fat-free beef broth	Lean roast lamb with mint
Cream of Wheat	Sliced white meat of chicken	jelly
Skimmed milk	Fat-free mashed potatoes	Parsley potatoes
2 slices toast	Green beans	Peas and carrots
Jelly	Enriched white bread	Asparagus salad
Decaffeinated coffee*	Jelly	Enriched white bread
	Canned peaches	Gelatin with fruit
	Skimmed milk	Tea
		Skimmed milk

DIET HIGH IN IRON

The foods highest in iron are liver, beef, veal, lamb, pork, turkey, chicken, oysters, enriched bread and cereals, eggs, peanut butter, dried navy and lima beans, soybeans, dried apricots, peaches, prunes figs, dates, raisins, and molasses.

SAMPLE MENU

Breakfast	Lunch	Dinner
Stewed prunes	Navy bean soup	Broiled liver with onions
Oatmeal	Chicken sandwich	Mashed potatoes
Cream	Carrot and raisin salad	Fresh broccoli
Poached egg	Citrus fruit cup	Tomato salad
Toast	Milk	Whole-wheat bread
Butter or margarine		Butter or margarine
Coffee		Date pudding
		Milk

BLAND DIET

A bland diet is moderately low in roughage and is mechanically, chemically, and thermally nonirritating. It contains fiber of a soft, nonirritating type as well as some residue from other sources, such as milk and milk products. The diet should contain generous amounts of milk and other protein foods to aid in counteracting gastric acidity. Three moderately small meals with between-meal feedings are the usual procedure. The bland diet is adequate if properly planned.

The following foods are included in bland diets of the traditional conservative type†:

Beverages   Milk, eggnog, vanilla milk shake, vanilla malted milk, Postum, decaffeinated coffee, weak tea

*Coffee is sometimes not permitted for patients with gallbladder disturbances.
†Many physicians today are using a much more liberal approach based on individual food tolerances and responses of each patient being treated. A background discussion of the history of peptic ulcer treatment and a comparison of the traditional and individual approaches may be found in Williams, S. R.: Gastrointestinal diseases. In Nutrition and diet therapy, ed. 3, St. Louis, 1977, The C. V. Mosby Co., pp. 532-536.

Bread	Day-old white bread, fine rye bread, toast, soda crackers
Cereal	Cream of Wheat, strained oatmeal, cornmeal, Cream of Rice, cornflakes, Rice Krispies, puffed rice, Corn Kix
Cheese	Cream cheese, cottage cheese, or mild American cheese when combined with potatoes, macaroni, or spaghetti
Dessert	Gelatin, plain bread pudding, plain tapioca pudding, plain rice pudding, junket, custard, plain cake, plain cookies, prune whip or apricot whip, and vanilla ice cream if eaten very slowly so that it is body temperature by the time it reaches the stomach
Eggs	Any way except fried
Fats	Cream and butter
Fruits	Canned peaches, pears, Royal Anne cherries, applesauce, baked apple without skin, canned apricots without skin, pureed prunes
Fruit juices	Prune juice, pear juice, peach juice, orange juice, grape juice (orange and grape juice should be taken at end of meal)
Meat, poultry, and fish	Beef, lamb, or veal (may be broiled, boiled, or baked), broiled crisp bacon, broiled liver, white meat of fowl (may be baked, boiled, broiled, or creamed), white-fish, salmon, or tuna
Potatoes	Potatoes (may be baked, boiled, buttered, mashed, or creamed)
Potato substitutes	Macaroni, spaghetti, noodles, or rice
Soups	Cream soups made from allowed vegetables, cream of rice or barley soup, cream of potato soup, strained cream of celery soup
Seasoning	Only salt in moderation
Sweets	Sugar, plain candies, honey and jelly in moderation, preferably at end of meal
Vegetables	Very young tender carrots, beets, string beans, wax beans, spinach, squash without seeds or skin, asparagus tips, peas (if not young and tender, must be strained)

In a bland diet, the following foods should be *avoided*.

High seasoned foods, especially with pepper

Meats with coarse fiber and tough gristle or meat juices

Fried foods

Any vegetables or fruits not on previous list

Foods containing much residue

Coffee, colas, or alcohol

SAMPLE MENU

Breakfast	Lunch	Dinner
Pear nectar	Roast beef	Cream of pea soup
Oatmeal	Browned potato	Breast of chicken
Soft-cooked egg	Buttered carrots	Baked potato with butter
Toast	White bread	Asparagus tips
Butter	Butter	Angel food cake
Decaffeinated coffee	Baked apple	Tea, weak
Milk	Tea, weak	Milk

LOW-RESIDUE DIET

A low-residue diet will leave a relatively small amount of residue, or indigestible material, in the colon. This type of diet is useful in colon and rectal surgery and in the treatment of diarrhea. This diet, as listed below, is deficient in vitamins.

The following foods are included in a low-residue diet.

Beverages	Cocoa, tea, coffee, strained fruit juices, carbonated beverages, milk
Bread and cereals	Melba toast, zwieback, white bread, white crackers, Cream of Wheat, strained oatmeal, rice, Rice Krispies, cornflakes, and puffed rice
Cheese	Cream and cottage, small amount of grated American cheese
Dessert	Simple puddings, gelatin, custard, sherbet, vanilla ice cream, plain cookies, angel food cake, and sponge cake
Eggs	Any way except fried
Fats	Butter, cream
Fruits	Applesauce, canned peaches, pears, Royal Anne cherries, pureed apricots, prunes, and plums, all fruit juices (orange juice may need to be strained)
Meat, poultry, and fish	Tender steaks, lamb chops, roast beef, roast lamb or veal, crisp bacon, ground beef patty, all fish, and white meat of fowl (all meats, fish, and poultry must be broiled, boiled, or baked)
Potatoes	Cooked in any way except fried
Potato substitutes	Broth soups containing noodles or rice, cream of potato,
Soups	cream of chicken, cream of asparagus, cream of tomato (all other soups must be strained)
Seasonings	Salt and pepper
Sugar	As desired
Vegetables	All vegetables (must be pureed), all vegetable juices

SAMPLE MENU

Breakfast	Lunch	Dinner
Strained orange juice	Strained vegetable soup	Chicken rice soup
Cream of Wheat	Broiled lamb chop	Chicken and noodle casserole
Cream	Baked potato	
Soft-cooked egg	Pureed string beans	Tomato juice
Toast	White bread	White bread
Butter	Butter	Butter
Jelly	Baked custard	Apricot puree
Coffee	Tea	Tea

MINIMUM-RESIDUE DIET

A minimum-residue diet is sometimes used after surgery on the lower part of the intestinal tract. This diet is below the recommended allowances in calcium and vitamin A and may be low in riboflavin.

The following foods are include in mimimun residue diets:

Beverages	Carbonated beverages, cereal beverages, coffee, tea
Bread	Toasted white bread, saltines, soda crackers
Cereal	Cooked refined rice, Cream of Wheat, strained oatmeal, Rice Krispies, puffed rice
Cheese	Cottage, cream
Dessert	Plain cakes, plain cookies, custards, gelatin, sherbet
Eggs	Cooked in any way except fried (scrambled eggs should be cooked in double boiler)
Fats	Butter, cream, fortified margarine
Fish or fowl	Broiled, boiled, or baked breast of chicken, broiled or baked fish
Fruits	Strained fruit juice, including 1 citrus fruit juice
Meats	Very tender beef, lamb, or veal (may be roasted, baked or broiled), broiled tenderloin, scraped steak
Potato substitutes	Macaroni, noodles, refined rice, spaghetti
Seasonings	Salt, spices in moderation
Soup	Bouillon, broth
Sweets	Honey, jelly, molasses, syrups, sugar, and candy that does not contain fruit or nuts
Vegetables	Tomato juice, carrot juice

The following foods should be *excluded* from minimum residue diets.

Milk and milk drinks	Any fruits or vegetables
Whole-wheat bread, quick breads	Fried foods
Whole-grain cereals	Potatoes, hominy, whole-grain rice

SAMPLE MENU

Breakfast	Lunch	Dinner
Strained orange juice	Broth with noodles	Tomato juice
Puffed rice	White meat of chicken	Small broiled tenderloin
Poached egg	Cottage cheese	Buttered rice
Melba toast	Melba toast	Melba toast
Butter	Butter	Butter
Jelly	Gelatin	Jelly
Cream	Tea	Angel food cake
Coffee	Plain cookies	Tea

HIGH-RESIDUE DIET

Recent studies in the incidence and treatment of colon diseases such as diverticulitis and colon cancer have related these intestinal problems to the increased use of refined foods in the urban diet. As a result, the treatment being used in some centers for diverticulosis is an increase in fiber and in residue foods such as whole grains and bran, rather than the traditional low residue diet therapy.

SODIUM-RESTRICTED DIET

The sodium-restricted diet is an allowance of food and drink in which the sodium content is limited to a specified amount.

Sodium is an essential element of the body. By osmotic pressure, it maintains the proper balance between the volume of intracellular and extracellular fluids.

A normal adult has about 50 liters of fluid in his body. Most of this fluid is within the cells, but about 15 liters are extracellular—the fluid surrounding the cells ("extra" means "outside of"). Sodium is present primarily in the extracellular fluid. Much less sodium (about one fourth as much) is present in the fluid within the cells.

This extracellular fluid has a constant composition of 3.3 grams of sodium per liter of fluid. Sodium is retained in the body only in solution; therefore, if larger than normal amounts of sodium are retained, larger than normal amounts of water will also be retained. A person in normal health is able to excrete the sodium not needed by the body primarily through the skin and also through the kidneys and bowels. However, in certain diseases too much sodium is retained, and as a result there is edema or an abnormal accumulation of extracellular fluids. Formerly, fluids were restricted for patients with edema, but this is no longer necessary if sodium is restricted instead.

Often a low-sodium diet is prescribed for a cardiac patient. However, whether or not the diet for this patient is low in sodium, it should be calculated to reduce the load on the heart. This is best accomplished by giving five or six small meals a day of easily digested foods, avoiding all bulky foods and gas-forming vegetables.

There has been some confusion in terminology resulting from the practice of using the words "salt" and "sodium" interchangeably. The confusion has resulted from the fact that such a large proportion of salt is sodium (46%). One-fourth teaspoon of salt contains approximately 450 mg. of sodium. The percentage of sodium is also high in baking powder, baking soda, and many other products used in processing foods. Natural foods contain less sodium than those that have been processed. Animal foods are higher in natural sodium than fruits and most vegetables. Some city water is very high in sodium, and this is a point to be considered in calculating a low sodium diet. Water softeners increase the sodium content of the water, and water containing a softener should not be used in preparing a low-sodium diet.

A normal person not on a restricted-sodium diet usually receives from 3,000 to 5,000 mg. of sodium a day. That is approximately twice as much as is needed by the body, but the excess is promptly excreted.

The amount of sodium in the diet is usually restricted to one of five different levels, the particular amount to be determined by the physician.

In the following meal plans for diets containing 2,000 to 3,000 mg., 1,000 mg., 800 mg., and 500 mg. of sodium, an allowance of 100 mg. has been made for 1 quart of water to be used for drinking purposes and for use in making beverages such as coffee and tea. On a 200 mg. sodium diet, distilled water should be used for drinking and in making beverages.

When the diet is "low in salt," requiring a mild sodium restriction (2,000 to 3,000 mg. sodium), the following dietary procedures are observed:

Food is cooked with a minimum of salt.
No salt is used at the table.
No highly salted foods are used.

No foods high in sodium are permitted.
Meat, broth, soups, and butter without salt are given.

When the sodium is restricted to 1,000 mg., the food is cooked without salt, and no foods high in sodium are permitted. The following meal plan is suggested:

Regular milk	1 pint
Unsalted egg	1
Unsalted meat	6 oz., cooked
Fruit (1 citrus)	As desired
Unsalted vegetables	3 servings
Unsalted bread and its exchanges	As desired
Regular bread	1 slice
Unsalted fats, sugar, and jelly that is free from sodium preservatives	

The same dietary procedures (food cooked without salt, and so on) are observed when the sodium is restricted to 800 mg. The following meal plan is suggested:

Regular milk	1 pint
Unsalted egg	1
Unsalted meat	6 oz., cooked
Unsalted vegetables	3 servings
Fruit (1 citrus)	As desired
Unsalted bread and its exchange	As desired
Regular bread	2 slices
Unsalted fats, sugar, and jelly that is free from sodium preservatives	

The same dietary procedures are again observed when the sodium is restricted to 500 mg. The following meal plan is suggested:

Regular milk	1 cup
Low-sodium milk	1 cup
Unsalted egg	1
Unsalted meat	6 oz., cooked
Unsalted vegetables	3 servings
Fruit (1 citrus)	As desired
Unsalted bread and its exchanges	As desired
Fats, sugar, and jelly that is free from sodium preservatives	

When the sodium is restricted to 200 mg., the same dietary procedures as for the previous sodium restrictions are observed. The following meal plan is suggested:

Low-sodium milk	1 pint
Unsalted egg	None (unless substituted for 3 oz. meat)
Unsalted meat	5 oz., cooked
Unsalted vegetables	3 servings
Fruit (1 citrus)	3 servings
Unsalted bread and its exchanges	6 servings
Fats, sugar, and jelly that is free from sodium preservatives	

Following is a list of foods that are allowed and those that must be avoided. All allowed foods must be prepared without the addition of salt or other seasoning containing sodium.

Foods allowed	Foods to avoid
Dairy products	
Whole milk	Cheese, other than low-sodium cottage cheese
Skim milk	Cultured buttermilk
Low-sodium milk	Sour cream or heavy sweet cream
Homemade ice cream made from eggs and milk allowance	(On 500 mg. sodium diet, 2 tbs. may be used; on 200 mg. sodium diet, none is used)
	Commercial ice cream
	(1/2 cup commercial ice cream may be substituted occasionally for 1 cup milk on 800 to 1,000 mg. sodium diets only)
Beverages	
Coffee	Cocoa, Dutch process
Decaffeinated coffee	
Postum	
Tea	
Hershey's cocoa	
Fruit juice	
Cola drinks	
Orange drinks	
Lemonade	
Orangeade	
Bread and cereals	
Unsalted bread	Regular bread unless doctor allows it
Unsalted matzoth	Quick-cooking cereals
Unsalted cooked cereal	Dry cereals not listed
Shredded wheat	Self-rising flour
Puffed rice	Salted or soda crackers
Puffed wheat	Pretzels
Unsalted cooked rice	
Desserts	
Custard or ice cream made at home from egg and milk allowance	Desserts prepared with salt, baking powder, baking soda, or egg white
Gelatin desserts made with plain gelatin and foods allowed	Commercial gelatin desserts
	Commercial ice cream

Foods allowed	Foods to avoid
Unsalted fruit pie or pudding made from foods allowed	Rennet desserts
Desserts prepared without salt, baking powder, baking soda, or egg white	
(¹/₂ cup commercial ice cream may be substituted for 1 cup milk occasionally on 800 to 1,000 mg. sodium diet)	

Eggs

Eggs in allowed amounts

Fats

Unsalted butter or margarine	Bacon fat
Cream, ¹/₃ cup daily (except on 200 mg. sodium diet)	Salted butter
	Salted margarine
Unsalted salad dressings	Salted salad dressings
Salad oil	
Unsalted shortening	

Fruits

All fruits except those listed to avoid	Cantaloupe, raisins, and dried figs (cardiac patients should avoid all raw fruits except citrus)

Meat, fish, and fowl

Beef	Brains
Lamb	Clams
Pork	Crab
Veal	Shrimp
Liver	Heart
Chicken	Kidney
Turkey	Lobster
Fresh oysters	Frozen fish
Fresh fish	Salted, smoked, or salted canned meat

Potatoes and potato substitutes

Potatoes, white	Hominy
Potatoes, sweet	Potato chips
Macaroni	
Spaghetti	
Homemade noodles	
Rice	

Soups

Unsalted cream soup made from milk allowance and allowed vegetables	Canned or condensed soups
Unsalted broth soups	

Sweets

Pure sugar candy	Candy, except that listed under *Foods allowed*
Honey	
Jam, jelly, or marmalade made without sodium benzoate	
Molasses	
Syrups, homemade	
Sugar	

Foods allowed	Foods to avoid

Vegetables
(All vegetables must be fresh, or canned without salt or other sodium product.)

Foods allowed	Foods to avoid
Asparagus	Celery
Beans, string, wax, and fresh lima	Beets
Broccoli	Greens—beet and dandelion greens, spinach,
Brussels sprouts	kale, and Swiss chard
Cabbage	Frozen peas
Carrots	Frozen lima beans
Cauliflower	Sauerkraut
Cucumbers	(cardiac patients should avoid broccoli,
Eggplant	Brussels sprouts, cabbage, cauliflower,
Endive	cucumbers, onions, green peppers, and
Green peppers	turnips)
Lettuce	
Mushrooms	
Onions	
Peas, fresh	
Pumpkin, fresh	
Squash	
Tomatoes	
Turnips	

Miscellaneous

Foods allowed	Foods to avoid
Hershey's chocolate	Regular catsup
Herbs	Chili sauce
Spices and vinegar in moderation	Gravy
Unsalted nuts	Prepared horseradish
Unsalted popcorn	Prepared mustard
Unsalted white sauce made with milk	Salted nuts
allowances	Olives
Unsalted catsup	Salted peanut butter
	Salted pickles
	Salted popcorn
	Relishes
	Salt
	Baking powder
	Baking soda
	Bouillon cubes
	Prepared salad dressings and sauces
	Chemically softened water

Many spices, herbs, and seasonings may be used to improve the flavor of low-sodium diets. The following list of flavoring aids may be used as desired on low-sodium diets:

Allspice	Cardamon
Almond extract	Chives
Anise	Cinnamon
Basil	Cloves
Bay leaf	Cocoa (not Dutch process)
Caraway	Curry

Dill	Pimiento
Garlic	Poppy seed
Ginger	Poultry seasoning
Horseradish (fresh)	Rosemary
Lemon juice or extract	Saccharin
Mace	Saffron
Maple extract	Sage
Marjoram	Savory
Mint	Sesame
Mustard, dry	Sucaryl, calcium
Nutmeg	Sugar, brown, in small amounts
Onion juice, fresh	Sugar, white
Orange extract	Tarragon
Oregano	Thyme
Paprika	Tumeric
Parsley	Vanilla extract
Pepper	Wine
Peppermint extract	

The following seasonings should not be used on low-sodium diets.

Bouillon cubes	Mustard, prepared
Catsup	Olives
Celery salt	Pickles
French dressing, commercial	Salt, plain or iodized
Garlic salt	Syrups, commercial
Mayonnaise, commercial	Worchestershire sauce
Meat sauces	

Questions on modifications of individual constituents

1. Plan a 1-day menu for a high-calorie diet and calculate the number of calories in the diet, using the table of food values in the Appendix.
2. List the foods that are emphasized on a high-protein diet. Plan a menu for one day for a person on a high-protein diet, and a menu for a person on a low-protein diet.
3. Plan a high-carbohydrate diet for 1 day.
4. What foods are restricted in quantity on a low-fat diet?
5. What foods are restricted in a minimum-fat diet?
6. Name five foods high in iron.
7. How does a bland diet differ from a regular diet?
8. What are the differences between a low-residue diet and a minimum-residue diet?
9. Plan a day's menu for a person on a low-residue diet, and one for a person on a minimum-residue diet.
10. Which two of the following desserts may be used on a low-protein diet: fruit cup, custard, geletin cubes with whipped cream, lemon pie?
11. Which two of the following foods are allowed on a low-residue diet: Cream of Wheat, cocoa, lettuce, creamed peas, buttered carrots, cherry pie?
12. What is the most important function of sodium in the body?
13. How is sodium concerned with the formation of edema?
14. What is the difference between salt and sodium?

15. What foods would you suggest for a restricted sodium diet?
16. Plan a menu for a 500 mg. sodium diet for 1 day.
17. Name five seasonings that could be used in preparing low-sodium diets, and name the foods on which they would be used.

Suggestions for additional study

1. Using the table of food values in the Appendix, calculate the number of grams of protein in the high-protein and low-protein diets you have planned.
2. List all the diets discussed in this chapter in which the following foods could be used: chicken-rice soup, white meat of chicken, tomato juice, pureed peas, beets, carbonated beverages, milk, ice cream, and vegetable soup.
3. Plan a 500 mg. sodium diet; prepare and eat the foods as planned for 1 day. What suggestions do you have for making the the food more palatable?
4. Make a study of the various herbs that may be used on the low-sodium diet and learn, by actually tasting, what flavor they give to the food by their use.

References

Bills, C. E., McDonald, F. G., Niedermeier, W., and Schwartz, M. C.: Sodium and potassium in foods and waters, J. Am. Diet. Assoc. **25**:304-314, 1949.

Division of Biology and Agriculture, National Academy of Sciences–National Research Council: Sodium restricted diets, publication no. 325, Washington, D.C., 1954, The Academy.

Williams, S. R.: Nutrition and diet therapy, ed. 3, St. Louis, 1977, The C. V. Mosby Co., Unit 4.

Williams, S. R.: Essentials of nutrition and diet therapy, ed. 2, St. Louis, 1978, The C. V. Mosby Co., Part 3.

16

Diseases of the gastrointestinal tract

The gastrointestinal tract comprises the stomach and the intestines and is one of the areas in which much of the treatment depends on supplying the correct diet for each particular type of gastrointestinal disturbance. The area is exposed to all kinds of dietary indiscretion, and it is affected by mental and emotional disturbances to a greater extent than are the rest of the organs involved in the processes of digestion and metabolism.

In the following paragraphs a few of the more frequent diseases of the gastrointestinal tract are discussed. To prevent any misunderstanding, it is necessary to review the meaning of a few terms at this point. "Dietary fiber" is used to describe a variety of the undigestible portions of common foods, including several different groups of material—cellulose, hemicellulose, lignin, and pectin. "Residue" is used to describe the form of the food as it reaches the large intestine. "Roughage" is used to describe the food before it enters the body. A so-called bland diet is a diet in which all foods that cause chemical, mechanical, or thermal irritation are avoided.

COLITIS

Colitis is an inflammation of the mucous membrane of the colon. There are three types of colitis: simple colitis, mucous colitis, and ulcerative colitis.

Simple colitis is characterized by spasmodic pain and alternating constipation and diarrhea. The patient is usually under tension, and faulty food habits and the use of laxatives and enemas may be involved. The low-residue diet described in Chapter 15 should be followed with an emphasis on protein foods for healing tissue. Cathartics are withdrawn, and constipation is relieved by taking agar, Metamucil, or some other soft, bulk-producing agent.

Mucous colitis is characterized by constipation and the passage of large quantities of mucus, usually preceded by abdominal pain. This type of colitis is usually found in neurotic persons who have a long history of constipation and the use of purgatives. The same type of diet should be used here as in simple colitis, and again, agar or some other soft, bulk-producing agent should be used to combat constipation.

Ulcerative colitis is an organic disease characterized by inflammation of the mucous membrane of the large intestine. At first the mucous membrane contains a large amount of tissue fluid and an unusual amount of blood and bleeds easily. The cause of ulcerative colitis is not known, but there are four possible causes: (1) microorganisms within the body, (2) inadequate amounts of vitamin B complex and complete proteins, (3) allergy, and (4) emotional disturbances. Once established, ulcerative colitis is usually chronic. As yet, no permanent cure has been found, but the disease can be temporarily arrested.

The dietary treatment for ulcerative colitis may be accompanied by bed rest and psychotherapy. In the acute stage, a liquid diet should be given. The diet following the acute stage should be the minimum-residue diet; as the patient improves, the low-residue diet may be given. As soon as safety allows, a bland high-protein, high-calorie diet should be given. The greater selection of foods serves to improve the patient's morale. The diet should also be high in vitamins and minerals. In addition to vitamins in the diet, vitamin supplements, especially vitamin B complex, should be given in double the normal amounts. Large amounts of vitamins are needed because of lack of absorption. The protein should be high because of the amount of protein lost in the feces and through hemorrhage. The diet should be low in fat, and the only fats used should be butter and cream. Supplementary iron should also be given, since anemia is frequently found in ulcerative colitis. Milk is usually not tolerated well. If the patient cannot take milk, a calcium supplement should be given.

The patient should eat three meals a day and have between-meal feedings. Adequate fluids must be taken in the amount of 6 to 8 glasses daily. Nervous strain, emotional tension, and fatigue should be avoided. If there is constipation, corrective medication should be taken only on the advice of a physician.

DIARRHEA

Diarrhea has various causes—the wrong foods, allergy, food poisoning, excessive use of cathartics, nervousness, or the presence of bacterial disease. It usually corrects itself if the cause is removed.

The fundamentals of the dietary treatment of diarrhea include the following:
1. Normal amounts of calories unless the patient is emaciated
2. High-calorie diet if emaciation is present
3. All of the necessary nutrients in adequate amounts
4. A diet high in vitamins to counteract lack of absorption
5. High-quality, well-prepared food attractively served
6. Food low in residue
7. Food chewed well before swallowed
8. Food intake for the day divided into six small feedings

If the feces show undigested starch, the patient should receive less starch and more protein, such as ground meat, broth soups, eggs, and milk. Pureed vegetables and a small amount of toast may also be served. Only small amounts of sweets are allowed. If there is meat fiber in the feces, the diet should be as low as possible in protein, and such foods as cereal gruels, toast, mashed potatoes, rice, bread with butter and jelly, and milk should be given. Applesauce or scraped apple may be given between meals since the pectin in apples tends to help in the treatment of mild diarrheas.

MALABSORPTION SYNDROME (SPRUE, CELIAC DISEASE)

Sprue is a general term given to intestinal malabsorption disorders. Fat, especially, is poorly absorbed. Thus, the characteristic diarrhea in sprue consists mainly of multiple foamy, bulky, greasy stools high in fat content. Adult nontropical sprue is similar in nature to childhood celiac disease.

A factor recently discovered to be important in the cause of sprue and celiac disease is *gluten*. Gluten is a protein found mainly in wheat, with some additional amounts in rye and oat. The gluten-free diet given in Table 16-1 has been widely used with marked improvement in symptoms.

Table 16-1. Gluten-free diet for nontropical sprue*

Characteristics

1. All forms of *wheat, rye, oat, buckwheat,* and *barley* are omitted except gluten-free wheat starch (Cellu Products Co.).
2. All other foods are permitted freely, unless specified otherwise by the doctor.
3. The diet should be high in protein, calories, vitamins, and minerals.

Foods	Allowed	Not allowed
Milk (2 glasses or more)	As desired	
Cheese	Any, as desired	
Eggs (1 or 2 daily)		
Meat, fish, fowl (1 or 2 servings)	Any plain meat	Breaded, creamed, or with with thickened gravy; no bread dressings
Soups	All clear and vegetable soups; cream soups thickened with cream, cornstarch, or potato flour only	No soup thickened with wheat flour; no canned soup except clear broth
Vegetables (2 servings of green or yellow daily, at least)	As desired, except creamed	No cream sauce or breading

*From Williams, S. R.: Nutrition and diet therapy, ed. 3, St. Louis, 1977, The C. V. Mosby Co.

Continued.

Table 16-1. Gluten-free diet for nontropical sprue—cont'd

Foods	Allowed	Not allowed
Fruits (At least 2 or 3 daily, including 1 citrus)	As desired	
Bread	Only that made from rice, corn, or soybean flour, or gluten-free wheat starch	All bread, rolls, crackers, cake, and cookies makde from wheat and rye; Ry-Krisp, muffins, biscuits, and waffles; pancake flour and other prepared mixes; rusks, zwieback, and pretzels; any product containing oatmeal, barley or buckwheat; any breaded food and food crumbs
Cereals	Cornflakes, cornmeal, hominy, rice, Rice Krispies, puffed rice, precooked rice cereals	No wheat or rye cereals, wheat germ, barley, buckwheat, kasha
Pastes		No macaroni, spaghetti, noodles, dumplings
Desserts	Gelatin, gelatin with fruit, ice and sherbet, homemade ice cream, custard, junket, rice pudding, cornstarch pudding (homemade)	Cakes, cookies, pastry; commercial ice cream and ice cream cones; prepared mixes, puddings; homemade puddings thickened with wheat flour
Beverages	Milk, fruit juices, ginger ale, cocoa (read label to see that no wheat flour has been added to cocoa or cocoa syrup); coffee (made from ground coffee), tea, carbonated beverages	Postum, malted milk, Ovaltine (read labels on instant coffees to see that no wheat flour has been added)
Condiments and sweets	Salt; sugar, white or brown; mollasses; jellies and jams; honey, corn syrup	Commercial candies containing cereal products (read labels)
Fats	Butter, margarine, oils	Commercial salad dressings, except pure mayonnaise (read labels)

CAUTION: Read labels on all packaged and prepared foods.

ACUTE ENTERITIS

Acute enteritis is a broad term signifying any inflammation of the bowel that is accompanied by diarrhea. It may be caused by toxins, bacteria, or anything that irritates the mucous lining of the intestines. If the case is acute, nothing should be given by mouth for 24 to 48 hours except small amounts of water or cracked ice. This can be followed by a liquid diet and a gradual return to a bland diet.

GASTRITIS

Gastritis is an inflammation of the mucous membrane of the stomach and may be either acute or chronic. It may be caused by dietary indiscretions, an excess of alcohol, overeating, or too many highly seasoned foods. If the condition is acute, a liquid diet must be given for the first 2 days, after which a small amount of cereal gruel or a small amount of milk may be given every hour. As the patient improves, the amounts may be increased and given every 2 hours. Gradually the diet may be increased by adding one low-residue food at a time until the patient is receiving a soft, bland diet.

In chronic gastritis, the cause should be determined, and the offending food or drink should be eliminated from the diet. The diet should consist of easily digested foods, such as those given in the bland diet.

CONSTIPATION

There are two kinds of constipation, atonic and spastic. In atonic constipation, the more common of the two, the walls of the intestines lack the necessary muscular tone to promote enough peristaltic action to push the food waste through the lower intestinal tract.

In spastic constipation, the descending colon is subject to contractions or spasms accompanied by pain, with narrowing of the descending colon to approximately one half to one third the diameter of the normal colon.

The causes of constipation are as follows:

1. Repeated failure to heed the normal urge for a bowel movement
2. Faulty dietary habits in which the person does not eat a sufficient amount of food containing roughage or fiber
3. Lack of exercise, which causes muscles to become weak and to lack tone
4. The use of laxatives, which builds up a dependence on their use and produces inflammation in the colon, often rushing the food on through the intestinal tract at a pace too rapid for complete absorption to take place
5. A limited intake of fluids, which results in dry, hard feces, making defecation difficult and painful

Atonic constipation

In regard to roughage or fiber, the foods that are of the most value in treating atonic constipation are whole grains, especially the bran portion, spinach, cabbage, cauliflower, asparagus, tomatoes, onions, and legumes. Fruits such as apples, pears, oranges, grapes, dried figs, raisins, and prunes are also valuable. Honey, too, has a mildly laxative effect. A glass of hot water with the juice of one-half lemon and 2 teaspoons of honey, taken on arising, and a 6-ounce glass of prune juice or a raw apple, taken on retiring, are beneficial. Prunes contain isatin, apparently a laxative factor. Milk is not a constipating food as such in most cases. Foods containing roughage should accompany protein foods such as milk, meat, poultry, fish, and eggs.

Spastic constipation

A person who has spastic constipation often responds to psychotherapy. There are numerous causes of spastic constipation, including excessive use of cathartics, condiments, or tobacco, eating foods high in fiber, such as bran, and drinking too much tea, coffee, or alcoholic beverages. Nervousness and tenseness are also contributory factors.

A person with this condition is not able to eat foods that have excess fiber, such as some raw vegetables and fruits, and therefore may tolerate better vegetables and fruits that have been strained or pureed. Fruits and vegetables are an important source of vitamins and minerals. In the beginning the minimum-residue diet should be given, and as the condition improves, the low-residue diet should be followed.

On arising in the morning, the patient may drink a glass of hot water with the juice of one-half lemon and 2 teaspoons of honey, and on retiring he should drink a 6-ounce glass of prune juice. Plain agar or Metamucil may be used if necessary to give further relief from the constipation. Plain agar is not a drug and can be taken in any reasonable amount. Through the absorption of water it gives soft bulk. It will not injure the mucous membranes of the stomach or intestines.

DIVERTICULITIS

Diverticulosis is the term used to indicate the presence of many small pouches, or pockets, that have formed along the intestinal tract, usually in the large colon. These diverticula usually occur in people past middle age. If one of these pockets becomes infected due to the accumulation of fecal matter, the conditions is called diverticulitis, and there is usually pain in the affected area. Sometimes perforation occurs, in which case surgery is indicated.

Following diverticulitis in which there has been no perforation, the patient should be given no food for the first day or so, after which he is given a liquid diet and then a minimum-residue diet. When the infection has subsided, a low-residue diet may be used briefly, but symptoms are relieved more over the long term by a generally high-fiber diet of about 8 to 10 grams of dietary fiber daily.

This more recent high-fiber diet for treatment of diverticulosis, rather than the traditional low-residue diet, has in most cases achieved remarkable improvement of symptoms. Residue in the colon seems to reduce the painful muscle contractions that are characteristic of the disease.

PEPTIC ULCER

Peptic ulcer includes both the gastric ulcer, which occurs in the stomach, and the duodenal ulcer, which occurs in the duodenum.

The objectives of diet in the treatment of an ulcer include the following:

1. To neutralize the acid gastric juice

2. To depress the flow of gastric juice
3. To promote healing of the ulcer by giving relief to the irritated area
4. To provide optimum nutrition as much as possible within the limitations of the diet

Characteristics of the traditional conservative ulcer diets are as follows:

1. The diet should be mechanically nonirritating. Foods should be bland and low in residue. Vegetables and fruits should be served in pureed form to eliminate the indigestible fiber. In the more acute stages, meat should be separated from the connective tissue by scraping it before it is cooked.

2. The diet should be chemically nonirritating. Excessively sweet or sour foods and highly seasoned foods should be omitted. Some other food items that have shown a stimulating effect on gastric secretions are coffee, tea, cola beverages, fried foods, condiments, and most spices. Alcohol and tobacco, while not classed as foods, are also restricted because of their stimulating effect on gastric secretions. The citrus fruit juices, although they are acid, may be used if they are diluted and taken after other food has been eaten. They are valuable because of their ascorbic acid content.

3. The diet should be thermally nonirritating. In other words, foods should not be extremely hot or extremely cold because of increased amount of acid is produced, and certain vascular changes incident to extremes of temperature are effected.

4. At first only foods that neutralize and inhibit acidity should be used in ulcer diets. Proteins and fats accomplish this purpose. The protein combines with the acid, reducing the acidity. Fats in the form of cream, butter, and egg yolk depress the secretion of the acids.

5. There should be frequent small feedings so that the stomach is never completely full or completely empty. The constant presence of some food in the stomach takes up the excess acid, which otherwise would cause pain and also delay the healing of the ulcer.

6. There should be gradual restoration to an adequate diet. The beginning ulcer diet is inadequate in some respects; therefore, it should be supplemented by vitamin concentrates and also by some form of iron. As the diet becomes more general, it is possible to keep it adequate by proper selection of foods.

The patient must understand that ulcers heal slowly and frequently return unless the diet is very carefully watched. With healing, the diet can perhaps be liberalized to a certain extent, depending upon individual food tolerances. (See footnote, p. 100, concerning bland diets in ulcer therapy.)

Beginning bland ulcer diet

The beginning ulcer diet is inadequate in iron, thiamine, niacin, and ascorbic acid. The diet should consist of hourly feedings from 7 A.M. through 10 P.M. They may consist of any one of the following mixtures:

1. 4 oz. half milk and half cream for 16 feedings
   Protein, 64 grams; fat, 230 grams; carbohydrate, 86 grams
   Calories, 2,670
2. 4 oz. milk and cream (3 oz. milk and 1 oz. cream) for 16 feedings
   Protein, 67 grams; fat, 154 grams; carbohydrate, 91 grams
   Calories, 2,018
3. 4 oz. skimmed milk for 16 feedings
   Protein, 70 grams; fat, 77 grams; carbohydrate, 96 grams
   Calories, 1,357
4. 4 oz. skimmed milk for 16 feedings
   Protein, 70 grams; fat, 2 grams; carbohydrate, 102 grams
   Calories, 706
5. 4 oz. milk, cream, lactose (3 pints milk, 1 pint cream, 6 level tbs. lactose for 16 feedings)
   Protein, 67 grams; fat, 154 grams; carbohydrate, 160 grams
   Calories, 2,294

After the first four days, the following foods may be substituted at 8 A.M., 12 noon, and 5 P.M.:

2 feedings: soft-cooked or poached egg
1 feeding: 6 tbs. strained oatmeal, Cream of Wheat, or Cream of Rice

As the patient improves, one of the following foods may be added to each of the hourly feedings: egg or cereal, as listed in the above diet, custard, milk toast, or plain pudding. This diet is still inadequate in the nutrients previously mentioned.

After about the third week, the foods in the following list may be added, one or two at a time. However, the diet will still be inadequate in iron, niacin, and ascorbic acid.

Beverages	Postum
Bread	Toasted enriched white bread
Cereals	None added
Cheese	Cream cheese or cottage cheese
Dessert	Plain rice pudding, prune whip, vanilla wafers, gelatin
Fats	Butter or margarine
Fruit	Strained applesauce
Eggs	Baked omelet, creamed or scrambled eggs prepared in a double boiler
Potatoes or potato substitutes	Potatoes (escalloped, mashed, baked, or creamed), noodles, white rice
Soup	Cream soups made with pureed asparagus, pureed carrots or peas, cream of potato soup, cream of rice soup, or cream of chicken soup

SAMPLE MENU

Breakfast	Lunch	Dinner
Poached egg	Cream of pea soup	Stained cream of asparagus
Toast	Baked potato with butter	soup
Half milk and half cream	Cottage cheese	Baked omelet
Strained applesauce	Melba toast	Mashed potatoes
	Butter	Melba toast
	Gelatin with whipped cream	Butter
	Half milk and half cream	Prune whip
		Half milk and half cream
10 A.M.	**3 P.M.**	**0 P.M.**
Cream of Wheat	Baked custard	Plain tapioca pudding
Half milk and half cream	Vanilla wafers	Half milk and half cream

Convalescent bland ulcer diet

As the patient improves further, he may progress gradually to the convalescent ulcer diet. It is possible to make this diet adequate in all the nutrients except ascorbic acid.

Foods included in the convalescent ulcer diet are the following:

Beverages	Cream, milk, half milk, and half cream, eggnog, vanilla malted milk, weak tea, decaffeinated coffee, Postum
Bread	White bread toasted, day-old white bread, white crackers
Butter	As desired
Cereals	Cream of Wheat, strained oatmeal, rice, Rice Krispies, corn-flakes
Cheese	Cottage, cream
Dessert	Custard, gelatin, junket, plain rice, cornstarch or tapioca pudding, angel food cake, sponge cake, hard white sugar cookies, vanilla wafers, arrowroot cookies, vanilla ice cream (eaten slowly)
Eggs	All forms except fried or scrambled in fat (scrambled eggs should be prepared over hot water)
Fish or fowl	Bake, boiled, and broiled fish, canned tuna, white meat of chicken or turkey that has been baked or boiled
Fruit	Applesauce, baked apple without skin, pureed apricots, pureed prunes, canned peaches, pears, Royal Anne cherries, very ripe bananas
Fruit juice	Orange juice ($1/4$ cup diluted with $1/4$ cup water), pear, peach, and apple juice, apricot nectar
Meat	Tender roast lamb, veal, and beef, broiled lamb chop, broiled chopped beef, small broiled tenderloin steak
Potato	Any way except fried
Potato substitutes	Rice, macaroni, spaghetti, or noodles
Soups	Cream soups made from strained vegetables as listed below, cream of chicken soup, cream of rice soup, cream of potato soup

Seasonings	Salt only
Sugar	As desired
Vegetables	Tender cooked asparagus tips, beets and carrots with skins removed, pureed string beans, spinach, peas, squash

Foods omitted from the convalescent ulcer diet are the following:

All fried, highly seasoned, and spiced foods	Catsup
Mustard	Horseradish
Vinegar	Pickles and relishes
Pepper	Meat soups and gravies, broths and bouillon
Smoked and preserved meat and fish	Coffee
Pork	Carbonated water
Raw fruit except ripe bananas, orange juice	Pastries
	Nuts
Raw vegetables	Raisins
Alcoholic beverages	Currants
	Candies

The following regulations should be observed:

1. The patient should receive supplementary feedings at 10 A.M., 3 P.M., and 8 P.M.

2. The patient should eat his meals slowly and chew them well.

3. The foods the patient eats should reach the stomach at body temperature.

4. During the first week, the varieties of food for any meal should be limited to four or less.

SAMPLE MENU

8 A.M.	10 A.M.	12 noon
Diluted orange juice	Eggnog	Cream of pea soup
Cream of Wheat	Crackers	Broiled lamb chop
Cream		Buttered carrots
Toast		Melba toast
Butter		Butter
Half milk and half cream		Canned pear
		Milk

3 P.M.	6 P.M.	9 P.M.
Baked custard	Potato soup	Gelatin with cream
Arrowroot cookies	Crackers	Angel food cake
Milk	Breast of chicken	Milk
	String bean puree	
	Melba toast	
	Butter	
	Prune whip	
	Milk	

Questions on diseases of the gastrointestinal tract

1. Why is diet an important factor in the treatment of gastrointestinal diseases?
2. Define residue.
3. What foods are included in the bland diet?
4. Name the three kinds of colitis. Describe each.
5. What are some of the possible causes of ulcerative colitis?
6. Outline the dietary treatment for ulcerative colitis.
7. What is the prognosis for ulcerative colitis?
8. What are the usual causes of diarrhea?
9. Which nutrients should be increased in cases of diarrhea and why?
10. Outline the total diet requirements in the treatment of diarrhea.
11. What diet should be given in the treatment of acute enteritis?
12. What is gastritis, and what diet is used in the treatment of an acute case?
13. Name the two kinds of constipation. Describe each.
14. What are some of the causes of constipation?
15. Give in detail the dietary management of atonic constipation.
16. What are some of the causes of spastic constipation?
17. What type of food should be used in the diet for spastic constipation?
18. What is diverticulitis?
19. Outline the diet for diverticulitis.
20. What are the objectives of the ulcer diets?
21. What is meant by "mechanically nonirritating"?
22. What are some of the foods that are chemically irritating to an ulcer patient?
23. List the spices and seasonings that may be used on the ulcer diet and those that may not be used.
24. Why and how should citrus fruit juices be used?
25. Why should extremes in hot or cold foods be avoided?
26. Why are milk, cream, and eggs so successful in the treatment of ulcers?
27. Why are small, frequent feedings necessary?
28. Plan a 1-day menu for a third-week ulcer diet.
29. Plan a 1-day menu for a convalescent ulcer diet.

Suggestions for additional study

1. Give some ways in which pureed vegetables can be made more acceptable to the patient.
2. Plan a menu for 3 days for a person with ulcerative colitis.

References

Schneider, M., Deluca, V., and Gray, S.: The effect of spice ingestion upon the stomach, Am. J. Gastroenterol. **26:**722-739, 1956.

Williams, S. R.: Nutrition and diet therapy, ed. 3, St. Louis, 1977, The C. V. Mosby Co.

Williams, S. R.: Essentials of nutrition and diet therapy, ed. 2, St. Louis, 1978, The C. V. Mosby Co.

17

Diseases of the liver and gallbladder

DISEASES OF THE LIVER

The liver is one of the largest and most important organs of the body concerned with the metabolism of food. It plays an essential role in the metabolism of carbohydrates, protein, and fat, especially during the changes the nutrients undergo after digestion.

1. It stores an appreciable amount of amino acids and releases them as they are needed. It has a part in synthesizing the plasma proteins—albumin, globulin, fibrinogen, and prothrombin. It maintains the proper ratio of albumin to globulin in the blood. It controls the concentration of amino acids in the blood. Any amino acids that are not needed for tissue building and repair are broken down by the liver. Approximately one half is converted into urea and excreted by the kidneys, and the other half is changed into glucose or fatty acids and used for heat and energy.

2. It converts the glucose resulting from the digestion of carbohydrates into glycogen and acts as a storehouse for most of the glycogen. It also converts the glycogen back to glucose as it is needed to maintain the blood sugar at its normal level.

3. It releases fatty acids through the bloodstream to the tissues of the body. Fats, which are not stored to any great extent in the healthy liver, impair the functional capacity of the liver if they are retained in excess.

4. It secretes bile, which is then carried through the main bile ducts to the hepatic duct and through the cystic duct to the gallbladder. The liver secretes 500 to1,000 ml. of bile daily. The bile contains the bile salts that make the utilization of fats possible and retard intestinal putrefaction. The bile salts are also necessary for the absorption of the fat-soluble vitamins. The bile carries the waste products, which are the result of hemoglobin destruction, to the duodenum, from where they proceed through the intestinal tract and are excreted in the feces.

5. It is a storehouse for about 95% of the body's supply of vitamin A and most of the vitamin D. It also stores small quantities of some of the other vitamins, principally vitamins K, E, and B_{12}.

6. It breaks down the worn-out blood cells from which iron is conserved and reused. However, the spleen also takes an active part in the degradation of these cells. Both iron and copper are stored in the liver. The presence of copper, although it is not a component of the red blood cells, is essential for their formation.

7. It is one of the organs responsible for producing antibodies that destroy harmful bacteria in the blood.

8. It synthesizes prothrombin and fibrinogen, which are necessary for the clotting of blood.

9. It is the chief source of plasma cholesterol, and it also plays an important part in removing cholesterol from the blood.

This list of important functions of the liver should make us aware of the essential part this organ plays in maintaining health. The objectives in dietary treatment of liver disturbances are to protect the liver against stress and to allow it to function as efficiently as possible.

Infectious hepatitis

The cause of infectious hepatitis is not definitely known, but it is believed that a virus is transmitted by the intestinal-oral route or by blood transfusions from a person who has had infectious hepatitis and still harbors the infection. Epidemics have been traced to contaminated food, water, and milk.

The chief symptoms of infectious hepatitis are jaundice and enlargement of the liver. The basis of treatment is bed rest and the proper diet. The diet should be high in protein and carbohydrate and low to moderate in fat, with calories ranging from 2,500 to 3,500 per day. An adequate or more than adequate storage of protein and carbohydrate in the liver protects it from further damage. A diet high in protein (100 to 125 grams) is necessary for repair of the damaged liver tissue. A generous amount of carbohydrate (300 to 500 grams) is given to provide for glycogen storage, to protect against toxins, and to raise the caloric content of the diet. A diet with a low to moderate fat content (50 to 90 grams) is recommended. Some fat is necessary in a high-protein diet, and fat-soluble vitamins are needed. Some fat is also needed to make the diet more palatable and therefore more acceptable to the patients. Fats should be limited largely to the more emulsified forms found in milk, cream, egg yolk, and butter.

At first the patient may not be able to eat solid food and should be given only liquids. However, the liquids given should be high in protein, carbohydrate, and calories and moderately low in fat. The following liquid diet contains 120 grams of protein, 300 grams of carbohydrate, 80 grams of fat, and 2,400 calories.

Breakfast	Lunch	Dinner
3/4 cup orange juice	Cream soup	Cream soup
1/2 cup cereal gruel	Gelatin	1/2 cup cereal gruel
1 glass whole milk	3/4 cup whole milk with 4 tbs. nonfat dry milk	3/4 cup whole milk with 4 tbs. nonfat dry milk
10 A.M.	**3 P.M.**	**9 P.M.**
High-protein eggnog	Chocolate milkshake	3/4 cup whole milk with 1/2 cup of vanilla ice cream and 2 tbs. of chocolate syrup
1 egg	3/4 cup whole milk	
4 tbs. nonfat dry milk	1/4 cup nonfat dry milk	
3 tbs. sugar	1 tbs. chocolate syrup	
3/4 cup whole milk	2 tbs. vanilla ice cream	
3 to 4 drops vanilla		
4 tbs. vanilla ice cream		

As the patient improves, the following diet may be given. There should be a gradual transition from the liquid diet to this diet, which contains 100 grams of protein, 260 grams of carbohydrate, 90 grams of fat, and 2,500 calories. Food for a day includes the following.

2 cups whole milk	3 servings vegetables (1 green or yellow)
2 cups skimmed milk	
7 oz. meat	2 servings fruit, 1 citrus
1 egg	1 serving fruit juice
6 slices bread	2 tbs. fat
1/2 cup cooked cereal or 3/4 cup dry cereal	2 tbs. sugar

Additional calories may be added by giving larger amounts of these foods.

Cirrhosis of the liver

Cirrhosis of the liver is caused by extreme malnutrition. Whether the condition is the result of alcoholism, chronic infectious hepatitis, or some other cause, the damage to the liver is equally serious.

If a diet that supplies the essential nutrients is given, some regeneration of the liver cells will occur unless there is already too much scar tissue in the liver.

During the acute stage, the patient should take only milk, cereals, milk toast, toast, cooked fruits, rice, and mashed potatoes. After the patient has shown some improvement, the diet should be high in calories, protein (100 to 125 grams), and carbohydrate (300 to 500 grams), and low to moderate in fat (50 to 90 grams), as for infectious hepatitis. If the disease progresses to a hepatic coma, the protein is restricted to tolerance levels (about 20 to 40 grams). In addition to these specifications, the diet should restrict sodium if there is any accumulation of fluids in the peritoneal cavity. It should also include foods high in vitamins, since the diet has been inadequate for some time in both vitamins and other nutrients. The fat-soluble vitamins would definitely be very low because the absorption of fats has been impaired. A complete vitamin supplement should be given, especially since the patient at first does not usually eat his food very well. Vitamin K is especially important because frequent hemorrhages in cirrhosis result from a lack of it. Vitamin C, or ascorbic acid, although a water-soluble vitamin, is needed in larger than normal quantities for its ability to improve the resistance of liver cells to certain toxins peculiar to the liver. The B vitamins should be added in larger than normal amounts to aid in metabolism of the increased amount of carbohydrate. Adding some brewer's yeast daily yields good results because of its high vitamin B and high protein content.

The person who is caring for the patient must be sure that the food is eaten. Sometimes the patient has anorexia and will not eat unless he is urged or is fed, but without a proper dietary intake, he cannot recover. Bland foods are usually better tolerated, and sometimes, as in infectious hepatitis, it is necessary to give all the nutrients in a liquid form. It may become necessary to resort to intravenous or tube feeding, especially for patients with varices in the esophagus.

DISEASE OF THE GALLBLADDER

Disease of the gallbladder can be caused by either infection or the presence of stones. The bile, which is manufactured in the liver, is collected by many small bile ducts and then travels through the hepatic and cystic ducts to the gallbladder. In the gallbladder the bile is concentrated and stored until needed. In the process of digestion, when fat enters the duodenum, it triggers the production of cholecystokinin, a hormone in the duodenum. This hormone then travels through the bloodstream to the gallbladder, causing the gallbladder to contract and to send bile down through the common duct to the intestines.

When the gallbladder becomes infected, it does not concentrate bile, but discharges a vastly different fluid. If stones have formed in the gallbladder, they may obstruct the outlet for the bile. There is pain when fatty foods are consumed, whether the trouble is caused by an infected gallbladder or gallstones.

In any type of gallbladder disturbance, the diet should be low in fat, especially in animal fat. The average patient can usually tolerate a small amount of fat in milk and butter. During the acute stage, the patient should take only milk, cereals, toast, milk toast, cooked fruits, rice, and mashed potatoes. After the acute stage, a more varied diet can be given. However, some patients with gallbladder disturbances may not tolerate spices, condiments, coffee, strong-flavored cooked vegetables, or raw vegetables. Eggs are not usually given, but sometimes they can be tolerated. All fried foods and pastries should be avoided.

Foods that may be used include the following:

Beverages	Skimmed milk or buttermilk made from skimmed milk, weak tea, fruit juices
Bread	Enriched white bread or whole-wheat bread as desired
Cereals	As desired except bran cereals
Eggs	One a day if tolerated (any way except fried)
Fat	Only 3 tsp. butter or fortified margarine a day

Fruits	Raw fruits such as ripe bananas and orange and grapefruit sections may be used; all other fruits must be cooked or canned
Meats, poultry, and fish	Lean meat, poultry, and fish (may be roasted, broiled, baked, or boiled without added fat, and all visible fat removed)
Soups	Any soups, except bean soups (no fats)
Vegetables	No raw vegetables except lettuce, no gas-forming vegetables such as broccoli, Brussels sprouts, cabbage, cauliflower, navy beans, or sauerkraut
Seasonings	Herbs and small amount of spices
Sugar	As desired

When gallstones are present, surgery is usually performed to remove them. However, it is best for the patient to remain on a low-fat diet for a while after surgery to allow the inflammation in the gallbladder area to subside.

Questions on diseases of the liver and gallbladder

1. Give one function of the liver in relation to amino acids.
2. What happens to the amino acids that are not needed for tissue building or repair?
3. What carbohydrate is stored in the liver, and how does the liver make use of it?
4. What happens to the fats that enter the liver?
5. What is the approximate daily secretion of bile from the liver?
6. Where does the bile go from the liver and through what channels?
7. What are the functions of the bile? Name three.
8. Name the two vitamins that are stored in the largest quantities in the liver.
9. What is the function of the liver in regard to the red blood cells?
10. What minerals are stored in the liver, and what is the function of each?
11. What role does the liver play in destroying harmful bacteria?
12. What are the objectives in dietary treatment of diseases of the liver?
13. What is believed to be the cause of infectious hepatitis?
14. What type of diet should be used in the treatment of infectious hepatitis?
15. Explain the reason for a high-protein and high-carbohydrate diet.
16. Why is it advisable to give some fat in the diet?
17. Plan a diet for 1 day for a patient with infectious hepatitis who is past the acute stage.
18. What is the direct cause of cirrhosis of the liver?
19. Describe the diet for a patient in the acute stage of cirrhosis of the liver.
20. When past the acute stage, what type of diet should a patient with cirrhosis of the liver have? When should sodium be restricted? Why should the diet be high in vitamins? Why is there a need for an increased amount of vitamins A and K, ascorbic acid, and the B vitamins? What feeding problems may arise?
21. What are the causes of gallbladder disturbances?
22. Trace the hepatic bile as formed in the liver until it reaches the intestines.
23. What hormone is involved in this process?
24. What type of diet is used in the treatment of gallbladder disturbances?

Suggestions for additional study

1. Plan a menu for 1 day for a patient in the acute stage of cirrhosis of the liver.
2. Make a drawing of the liver, showing the location of the gallbladder, the cystic duct, and the hepatic duct.

References

Kramer, P., and Caso, E. K.: Is the rationale for gastrointestinal therapy sound? J. Am. Diet. Assoc. **42:**505, 1963.

Williams, S. R.: Nutrition and diet therapy, ed. 3, St. Louis, 1977, The C. V. Mosby Co.

Williams, S. R.: Essentials of nutrition and diet therapy, ed. 2, St. Louis, 1978, The C. V. Mosby Co.

18

Diseases of the urinary tract

The kidneys are responsible for maintaining the normal composition of the blood. Here the blood is filtered and the waste products are excreted in the urine. Most of the waste products in the blood, except carbon dioxide, that result from the metabolism in the body are eliminated through the kidneys.

The two kidneys together contain approximately 2 million nephrons. Each of these nephrons contains a glomerulus, the filtering device of the kidneys. The blood plasma enters the glomeruli and is filtered. This filtrate is the same composition as blood except that it contains almost no protein. The glomeruli are attached to a tubule into which the filtrate passes. It then passes on through the collecting tubules into the pelvis of the kidney. The resulting fluid is urine, and it contains about 5% solids, the rest being water.

This phase of the kidney function is important, for it is in these tubules that the filtrate is divided and the part of the filtrate that is to be retained in the body is reabsorbed by the blood.

This reabsorption into the blood is not merely a return of the filtrate to the blood plasma; many changes in composition have been brought about by the tubules. The various chemicals that are needed by the body are taken from the filtrate and put back into the blood for use by the body, In fact, the final product of excretion, which is urine, is very different in both volume and composition from the filtrate as it comes from the glomerulus.

This is the means by which the body maintains the proper balance of sodium and potassium salts in the cells and in the spaces around the cells. It is also the way in which the body can discard excess salt and urea, the principal waste products of protein.

From the pelvis of the kidney, urine is passed through the ureters into the bladder, from which it will be eliminated. The normal amount of urine excreted daily is from 1 to 2 liters. Normal urine contains large amounts of urea, and if for any reason urea is not completely eliminated, it will be found in abnormal quantities in the blood. It is normal for blood to contain some urea.

NEPHRITIS

Nephritis is the term used to signify inflammation or degeneration of the kidney and its functions. It includes both acute and chronic glomerulonephritis, nephrosclerosis, and nephrosis. Although the basal metabolic rate does not change in nephritis, many times the patient's nutritional needs do increase because of the loss of food and water that occurs in vomiting and because of the loss of protein in the urine.

There is also often considerable loss of protein as a result of toxic destruction and loss of large quantities in the urine. The amount of protein in the diet should be limited to the amount needed to replace the tissue protein plus the amount of protein lost in the urine. The protein ingested should be of high biological value in order to be usable for tissue synthesis. Any protein in excess of the necessary amount will increase the work required of the already damaged kidneys.

The normal amounts of carbohydrates and fats are used in the diet of patients with nephritis because they put no strain on the kidneys.

Acute glomerulonephritis

In nephritis various parts of the nephron may be affected, but it is most often the glomeruli that are involved. The cause of acute glomerulonephritis is believed to be bacterial invasion, usually from a streptococcal infection. It is often the result of infectious childhood diseases such as scarlet fever or pharyngitis, and it may occur some time after the intitial infection. Streptococci do not lodge in the kidney but elsewhere in the body. Evidently, they produce a circulating toxin that is the active agent in glomerulonephritis.

The disease generally affects young children; approximately 50% of the patients are under 10 years of age. Most of them recover completely.

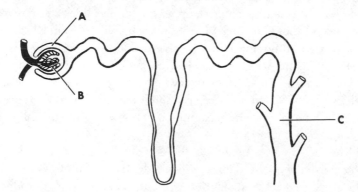

Fig. 3. A nephron. **A,** Glomerulus; **B,** glomerular capillaries; **C,** collecting duct.

In the acute stage the general nutrition of the patient will be sustained within limits of individual tolerance. If there is nausea and vomiting, the patient should be given lemonade, fruit juices, ginger ale, and tea, but no more than 1 quart of fluid per day should be given. After a few days milk, cereals, toast with jelly, and fruits may be added. When the patient has improved and has no more nausea or vomiting, he can be given an essentially normal diet, with the protein limited to between 45 and 50 grams and derived primarily from complete proteins. It is important that carbohydrates and fats be given in sufficient amounts to prevent the protein from being used for energy needs. Sodium should be restricted to 500 to 1,000 mg. if there is edema. The following diet contains 45 to 50 grams of protein and 1,550 calories.

2 cups milk	1 small potato
2 oz. meat or 1 egg and 1 oz. meat	2 servings other vegetables (1 green or yellow)
4 slices bread	3 servings fruit (1 citrus)
1/2 cup cooked cereal or 3/4 cup dry cereal	2 tbs. butter or fortified margarine
	7 tsp. sugar or jelly

These foods in the amounts given are to be eaten daily.

This diet is inadequate in niacin and iron. After the first 3 or 4 weeks, depending on the progress of the patient, the protein may be gradually raised to 80 to 90 grams. If the urinary output is increased, the fluids may be increased up to 1 1/2 quarts daily. The sodium can also be increased to include a little salt in the preparation of the food. Four ounces of meat and 1 cup of milk may be added to this diet to make 80 grams of protein and 2,000 calories. With these additions the diet will be adequate in niacin and iron.

Chronic glomerulonephritis

Chronic glomerulonephritis may occasionally follow an attack of the acute form. The patient sometimes has advanced chronic glomerulonephritis before there are any symptoms. Then vague symptoms, such as headaches, polyuria, and frequent urination at night, appear, later becoming more severe.

The diet should be high in protein, carbohydrate, and fat. Sodium may need to be restricted, but fluids may be given as desired.

Protein is needed for the repair of body tissues. The wear and tear on the body tissues continues in a person who is ill—perhaps even more so than in the well person, since there is usually some toxic destruction of protein in severe illness. Some physicians recommend the normal amount of protein plus the amount lost in the urine.

The carbohydrate content of the diet should be high in order to prevent the protein from being used for energy needs. If either dietray protein or body protein has to be broken down to provide energy, the waste product urea is then excreted through the kidneys, which increases the work load of the kidneys.

The fat content of the diet may also be high for the same reason unless the patient is troubled with anorexia. The fats used should be the emulsified fats, such as those found in egg yolk, butter, and cream.

If edema is present, sodium will need to be restricted to between 800 and 1,000 mg. This would mean that no salted foods or foods high in sodium would be used. No salt substitutes should ever be used unless ordered by the physician.

Fluids are not restricted, because the kidney is not able to concentrate the urine. Usually 1 to 2 quarts of liquids will be sufficient to satisfy thirst and to allow the excretion of solid waste products with a minimum amount of work for the kidney. In the case of fever or vomiting, more fluids may be required.

Nephrosclerosis

Nephrosclerosis is usually found among older people. It involves the circulatory system and thus impairs the kidneys. Symptoms usually include hypertension, changes in the retina, urea nitrogen retention in the blood, and sometimes albumin in the urine.

The protein in the diet should be maintained at the normal level if possible. When the blood urea nitrogen becomes excessively high, it indicates that the kidneys can no longer eliminate waste satisfactorily. In that case the protein should be restricted to 45 to 50 grams, as outlined in the diet for the treatment of acute glomerulonephritis. As much as possible of the 45 to 50 grams of protein should come from complete proteins. In more advanced conditions the protein may have to be limited to 25 to 35 grams. Carbohydrates should furnish more than half of the total calories. A part of the fat should be in the form of butter and cream. Milk should be included. Plenty of fruits and vegetables should be included because of their vitamin and mineral content, as well as for their base-forming properties. Condiments or alcoholic beverages are usually restricted. Only one cup of tea or coffee a day should be permitted. Foods should be bland. A reasonable amount of salt may be added to the food when it is cooked, but no salt should be added at the table, and no extremely salty foods should be served.

Moderate exercise such as walking or playing golf may be taken if the patient is able.

Nephrosis

The cause of nephrosis is not definitely understood. It is distinguished by the deterioration of the glomeruli and the tubules and also by the absence of hypertension, blood in the urine, anemia, retention of nitrogen, or cardiac involvement. There is severe depletion of serum proteins, as well as a tendency toward polyuria and edema.

In the dietary treatment of nephrosis, the protein should be high enough to furnish building material for body tissue and to replace the protein lost in the urine. The carbohydrate must be high enough to prevent the protein from being used to supply energy needs.

The beginning diet must provide 1,500 to 1,800 calories and furnish 50 to 60 grams of protein. Later the diet should be increased to 80 to 125 grams of protein and to 2,200 calories to keep pace with the patient's activity. No salt should be added to the food after it comes to the table, and if the patient has edema, the food must be prepared without salt.

UREMIA

In uremia, urea nitrogen is retained in the blood in abnormal amounts. It can result from nephritis, heart failure, extensive burns, toxemia of pregnancy, and any other organic disturbance that can cause an injury to the kidneys.

In uremia, the waste products are no longer excreted from the body. Nitrogenous products, especially urea, are abnormally retained in the body, and acidosis is usually present.

A patient with uremia should be allowed to have any foods that he can tolerate, but because of anorexia and vomiting, he will usually take only a few fruit juices or ginger ale at the beginning stage. He should be encouraged to take only foods or beverages that are principally carbohydrates and fats, since the metabolism of carbohydrates and fats does not involve any work on the part of the kidneys. Emergency measures, such as the butter-sugar diet originiated by Borst, have been used to furnish calories only. This diet consists of 200 grams of unsalted butter and 200 grams of sugar. The butter and sugar are made into balls and given to the patient at the meal hour.

More recently, a diet for uremic patients has been outlined by an Italian physician, Giovannetti, and used successfully in modified form in England and the United States. The modified Giovannetti diet allows 20 grams of protein composed of essential amino acids and ample carbohydrate for energy needs. Thus the excess urea and other nitrogenous materials are used by the body to make its needed nonessential amino acids.*

RENAL STONES

Renal stones are usually caused by chemical changes in the urine. Abnormal secretions from other organs in the body may affect the normal chemistry of the urine. Some persons have an obscure tendency to form stones in apparently normal urine, which is slightly acid.

There are three main kinds of renal stones: calcium phosphate, uric acid,

---

*An outline of the modified Giovannetti diet (basic food plan and food exchange lists) may be found in Williams, S. R.: Nutrition and diet therapy, ed. 3, St. Louis, 1977, The C. V. Mosby Co., pp. 587-592.

and calcium oxalate. A fourth, rare form is that of cystine stones, caused by a genetic disease. Calcium stones develop in alkaline urine; uric acid stones develop in urine that is too acid.

The diet prescribed in the treatment of calcium phosphate stones should be of predominately acid ash foods, which, of course, would also make it low in calcium. The low-calcium, acid ash foods are eggs, meats, fish, poultry, bread, cereals, corn, cranberries, plums, prunes, and rhubarb. They should be eaten liberally, and other foods such as milk, vegetables, and fruits should be used only in such amounts as are necessary for good nutrition.

The diet in the treatment of uric acid stones should be low in purines. This means that meats, poultry, and fish should be rigidly restricted to only 2 ounces a day. The following meats, meat products, and fish must be omitted entirely: anchovies, broth, bouillon, gravies, kidney, liver, meat extracts, roe, sardines, and sweetbreads. Only one of the following vegetables may be eaten daily: asparagus, beans (kidney, lima, or navy), lentils, mushrooms, peas, and spinach. Bread, cereals, cheese, eggs, fruit, milk, sweets, and other vegetables may be used freely.

The dietary treatment for calcium oxalate stones consists of the restriction of all foods high in calcium and in oxalates. Spinach, potatoes, beans, endive, tomatoes, dried figs, plums, strawberries, cocoa, coffee, and tea are foods that are high in oxalates and should be omitted from the diet. Foods that contain only a small amount of oxalates and may be used in reasonable amounts are bread, muscle meats, liver, sweetbreads, and cereals. Foods containing little or no oxalate that may be used in the diet freely are milk, cheese, eggs, butter and other fats, peas, rice, cabbage, cauliflower, asparagus, mushrooms, apricots, grapes, and melons.

An acid ash, low-purine, or low-oxalate diet is ineffective in removing stones that are already formed, but they can reduce the probability that stones will recur. The diet should be adequate and well balanced and contain sufficient protein to meet normal requirements. Water should be taken freely to prevent urine that is too concentrated.

Questions on diseases of the urinary tract

1. What is the function of the kidneys?
2. How many nephrons are in the kidneys?
3. What is the function of the glomeruli?
4. How does the composition of the filtrate compare with the composition of blood?
5. What is the percentage of solids in urine?
6. Trace the filtrate from the time it leaves the glomeruli until it becomes urine in the pelvis of the kidney.
7. What is the principal waste product of protein?
8. How does the urine reach the bladder?
9. What is the amount of urine normally excreted in a day?
10. What happens if the urea is not completely eliminated by the kidneys?

11. What is nephritis?
12. Through what channels is protein lost in nephritis?
13. What determines the amount of protein that should be in the diet in the treatment of nephritis?
14. Why is the amount of protein limited?
15. Why is the normal amount of carbohydrate and fat used in the diet for nephritis?
16. What is believed to be the cause of acute glomerulonephritis?
17. What age group does acute glomerulonephritis usually affect?
18. Discuss the diet in the treatment of acute glomerulonephritis.
19. Why should the diet for chronic glomerulonephritis be high in protein, carbohydrate, and fat? How would the presence of edema alter the diet? Why are fluids not restricted?
20. What age group does nephrosclerosis usually affect? When should protein be restricted to 45 to 50 grams a day and why? What percentage of the diet should be carbohydrate? What other specifications are included in regard to the diet?
21. What are the symptoms of nephrosis? How much protein and how many calories should be in the beginning diet, and how much should they be increased later on?
22. What are some of the causes of uremia? Why is the patient given principally carbohydrates and fats? What is the Borst diet?
23. Name the three main kinds of renal stones and describe the diet that should be given in the treatment of each.

Suggestions for additional study

1. Write a menu for 1 day for a 45- to 50-gram protein, 1,000 mg. sodium diet.
2. Plan a menu for 1 day for the following diets: (a) an acid ash diet, (b) a low-purine diet, and (c) a diet low in oxalates.
3. Trace the route taken by the blood plasma from the glomeruli to the bladder.

References

Williams, S. R.: Nutrition and diet therapy, ed. 3, St. Louis, 1977, The C. V. Mosby Co.

Williams, S. R.: Essentials of nutrition and diet therapy, ed. 2, St. Louis, 1978, The C. V. Mosby Co.

19

Diseases of the blood

The normal person has about 5 to 6 quarts of blood that travel the circuit of the vascular system in less than 30 seconds. The average number of red blood corpuscles in men is 5 million per cubic millimeter and in women, 4.5 million per cubic millimeter.

Blood consists of plasma, in which are suspended the erythrocytes, leukocytes, and platelets. The life of the erythrocyte, or red blood cell, is approximately 90 to 100 days, after which the old cell is destroyed and a new one is formed. The old red blood cell is usually destroyed in the spleen; the iron is saved for further use, and the remainder of the red blood cell is excreted. The red blood cell contains hemoglobin, which is made up of heme, a nonprotein iron compound, and globin, a protein. Iron is the oxygen-carrying element of the blood. The leukocytes, or white blood cells, act as scavengers and help resist infections. When the invading bacteria overcome them, the dead bodies of the leukocytes, or white blood corpuscles, collect in the form of pus, which causes an abscess if there is no outlet for it. The platelets have a part in the clotting process.

The functions of the blood are as follows:

1. It transports the end products of digestion from the digestive tract to the tissues of the body. It also carries oxygen from the lungs to the body tissues.
2. It carries the waste products of the body to the kidneys, lungs, skin, and intestines.
3. It carries the hormones to their target organs.
4. The white blood cells act as protection against disease.
5. It helps to regulate the body temperature.
6. It is essential for maintaining acid-base and water balance in the body.

ANEMIA

Anemia is a condition in which there is a reduction in the amount and size of the red blood corpuscles or in the amount of hemoglobin, or both. The symptoms of anemia are general weakness, poor appetite, pallor, fatigue, and increased sensitivity to cold. In more advanced conditions, gastrointestinal disturbances and difficult breathing occur.

The anemias are divided into the following three general classifications: (1) anemias due to loss of blood, called hemorrhagic anemia, (2) anemias due to the nutritional deficiency of iron or protein or the lack of absorption of these nutrients, called nutritional or iron deficiency anemia, and (3) anemia due to deficient formation of red blood cells in the bone marrow, called pernicious anemia.

Anemias due to loss of blood

Loss of blood occurs in excessive bleeding from an injury or from an abnormal condition within the body that results in a loss of blood volume. The body replaces the loss in volume with water, and in a normal person, the system automatically replaces the lost iron and other substances from the reserve in the body. However, a better than adequate amount of protein and iron in the diet will hasten the process. If the blood loss is large, a blood transfusion is advised.

Anemia often occurs in adolescent girls who experience excessive menstruation and whose diet is insufficient in protein and iron.

Nutritional anemias

Deficiency in iron. The adult body contains about 3 to 4 grams of iron, which is slowly absorbed from the food in the small intestine and passes in the blood to the bone marrow. There it is used in the manufacture of red blood cells. If there is a reduced amount of iron in the blood, the oxygen-carrying capacity is lessened.

The best answer to the problem of iron-deficiency anemia is prevention from fetal life onward. This means that during pregnancy the mother must have an adequate intake of iron (18 mg.) daily. This will ensure an adequate storage of iron in the fetus, which will meet the need for iron for the first 5 or 6 months of the infant's life, after which foods high in iron, such as egg yolk, should be added to the milk diet.

Throughout life all persons should be certain of receiving an adequate intake of iron, which is 10 mg. for men and 18 mg. for women. Additional iron (total of 18 mg.) is necessary for adolescent girls and women throughout their reproductive years because of menstruation and child-bearing demands. Adolescent boys should receive 18 mg. of iron daily because of rapid growth.

Deficiency in protein. Diets high in iron but inadequate in protein will not rebuild the red blood cells. When the amount of protein in the blood is reduced by hemorrhage, extensive burns, or pathological disturbances, the normal exchange of fluids between the blood vessels and the peritoneal cavities is lessened, and edema results.

Lack of absorption. In certain pathological conditions, iron is not properly utilized. Dietary iron must be changed in form through acid reduction before it can be absorbed. Thus, absorption of iron is facilitated by an acid medium. Iron absorption is aided by such agents as ascorbic acid (vitamin C). Most of the iron is absorbed in the duodenum, the first portion of the small intestine. This is because the gastric juice is acid and remains somewhat acid when it first enters the intestinal tract. Therefore, a person who has low gastric acidity needs both hydrochloric acid and iron supplements. The usual iron supplement given is ferrous sulfate, taken after each meal. It is less likely to upset the stomach if it is given following a meal.

The diet should be high in iron (20 to 25 mg.) and high in protein (100 to 150 grams). A diet high in iron but low in protein will not promote regeneration of hemoglobin. Liver is the most effective food in stimulating the production of blood. Liver once a week and lean meat and eggs daily are good sources of both iron and protein. Whole-grain or enriched bread and cereals, legumes, green leafy vegetables, and dried fruits are good sources of iron. The diet should also be high in vitamins, especially B complex and ascorbic acid. Insufficient calcium and vitamin D also interfere with proper utilization and storage of iron.

Pernicious anemia

Pernicious anemia is characterized by the deficient formation of red blood cells in the bone marrow. The cells become large and fewer in number. These large, immature red blood cells are called macrocytes. Normally, red blood cells are not released from bone marrow until they are mature. However, when the bone marrow becomes crowded with abnormal immature cells, they are released into the blood.

The symptoms of pernicious anemia are gastrointestinal disturbances, sore mouth, low gastric acidity, loss of appetite, neurological disturbances, and pain in the abdominal region.

The cause of pernicious anemia is the lack of the intrinsic factor in the gastric juice, which is essential for the absorption of vitamin B_{12}. Vitamin B_{12} is stored in the liver until needed by the bone marrow for maturing red blood cells. However, even though there is insufficient absorption of vitamin B_{12}, the liver is a sufficiently concentrated source of the vitamin to permit some absorption to take place without the intrinsic factor, thus protecting the nervous system from further damage.

In pernicious anemia, vitamin B_{12} is absorbed much better if it is given parenterally. When it is given by mouth, it is inadequately used because it has to pass through the gastrointestinal system, where there is inefficient absorption.

Formerly, liver extracts were given parenterally and achieved good results. However, the use of vitamin B_{12} has superseded the administration of liver extracts. Folic acid also helps in the treatment of pernicious anemia, but it should not be used as the only medication. It relieves some of the symptoms but does not improve the neurological disturbances.

The diet should be high in calories and protein. The diet should be high in carbohydrate in order to bring the weight up to normal and spare the protein for blood regeneration. The fat content should be low and made up largely of emulsified fats. The vitamins and minerals should also be increased. Iron supplements are usually given. Copper must also be present, but if an adequate diet is eaten, there will be sufficient copper. The consistency of the diet depends on the condition of the patient. If there is anorexia and perhaps soreness in the mouth, the beginning diet must be liquid. The patient will usually take liquids even though he has no desire for food. As the patient improves, the diet can be gradually changed to soft foods and a little later to regular foods.

After recovery, a patient with pernicious anemia must receive maintenance therapy of vitamin B_{12} injections for the rest of his life.

LEUKEMIA

Leukemia is characterized by a great excess of white blood cells that crowd out the red blood cells. There is enlargement of the spleen or lymphatics, or there are changes in the bone marrow.

Many times a patient with leukemia has a poor appetite, and frequent feedings are usually necessary. As a rule, the patient is weak and often has lesions in the mouth that make eating difficult. In this case he should be given soft foods that will not require much chewing. The foods given must not be highly spiced and must be neither too hot nor too cold. The foods that are the most acceptable are very tender meat, poultry, or fish, mashed potatoes, soft-cooked eggs, milk, and strained vegetables and fruits.

If cortisone or ACTH is used in the treatment, the diet will need to be low in sodium, since these medications tend to increase the reabsorption of sodium by the kidneys.

Current chemotherapy with various anti-cancer drugs has proved increasingly effective in controlling the disease process. However, optimal nutritional support in protein, calories, vitamins, and minerals must be provided throughout for successful therapy.

Questions on diseases of the blood

1. How much blood is present in the normal person?
2. What is the average red blood cell count for men? For women?
3. What three kinds of cells are found in the blood plasma?
4. What is the approximate life of the erythrocyte, and what happens when the cell is destroyed?
5. What is the composition of hemoglobin?
6. What is the function of iron in the blood?
7. What is the function of leukocytes? Of platelets?

8. List three functions of blood, excluding the individual functions of iron, leukocytes, and platelets.
9. What is anemia? List some of the symptoms.
10. Name the three types of anemia discussed in this chapter.
11. What are the possible causes of anemias due to loss of blood?
12. What deficiencies are responsible for nutritional anemia?
13. What is the normal content of iron in the adult body?
14. What are some of the causes of iron deficiency anemia?
15. Give in detail the diet for nutritional anemia.
16. What vitamins and what minerals, in addition to iron, are needed for regeneration of the blood?
17. What are the characteristics of pernicious anemia?
18. What is the cause of pernicious anemia?
19. What role does vitamin B_{12} have in the treatment of pernicious anemia, and how should it be administered?
20. Outline the dietary treatment for pernicious anemia.
21. Is there a permanent cure for pernicious anemia?
22. What is leukemia, and what are the symptoms for this type of blood disease?

Suggestions for additional study

1. Plan a day's menu for nutritional anemia and the same for pernicious anemia.
2. Circle the following foods that are high in iron: milk, eggs, whole-wheat bread, watermelon, tomatoes, navy beans.
3. Check the answer that correctly describes the diet for the treatment of nutritional anemia:
    a. High-caloric, low-protein, high-fat, high-iron, high–vitamin B complex, low–ascorbic acid, low-calcium, high–vitamin D.
    b. High-calorie, high-protein, low-fat, high–vitamin B complex, high–ascorbic acid, high–vitamin D, high-calcium, high-iron.
    c. High-calorie, high-protein, low-fat, high–vitamin K, low–ascorbic acid, high–vitamin D, low-calcium.

References

Williams, S. R.: Nutrition and diet therapy, ed. 3, St. Louis, 1977, The C. V. Mosby Co.

Williams, S. R.: Essentials of nutrition and diet therapy, ed. 2, St. Louis, 1978, The C. V. Mosby Co.

20

Diseases of the cardiovascular system

Cardiovascular diseases are responsible for approximately 50% of the deaths today. This is due partly to the fact that people in general are living longer and reaching the age at which degenerative diseases become more prevalent. Also, many people become obese in middle age, which makes them more susceptible to cardiovascular disturbances. Heart damage as a result of previous undiagnosed rheumatic fever is a contributing factor in the increasing death rate from cardiovascular diseases. Some persons with rheumatic heart disease and some with congenital heart disease have been restored to more active life by heart surgery.

The objectives in the dietary treatment of patients with heart disease are as follows:

1. To provide an adequate diet if the patient's condition permits
2. To prevent the patient from eating bulky or gas-forming foods that distend the stomach and exert pressure against the heart
3. To reduce the patient's weight to normal if he is overweight or to slightly below normal if he is not overweight, which permits the heart freer movement and lowers metabolism, thereby furnishing less stimulus to the heart
4. To prevent edema
5. To reduce the risk of atherosclerosis by lowering the number of circulating blood lipids

There are two types of cardiac disturbances: *functional* and *organic*. In the functional type, disturbances in the rate and regularity of the heartbeat are present. Often there are pains in the heart. The principal cause is infection; however, frequently it is due to psychological mechanisms.

The organic types of cardiac disturbances, which include rheumatic heart disease, pericarditis, coronary occlusion, angina pectoris, cardiac failure, atherosclerosis, and hypertension, are discussed separately on the pages that follow.

RHEUMATIC HEART DISEASE AND PERICARDITIS

Acute cardiac infection may result from rheumatic fever, or it may occur in pericarditis, which is inflammation of the membrane that encloses the heart. The objective of the diet should be to provide adequate nourishment with the least possible exertion on the part of the patient. Liquid and semiliquid foods such as milk, milk toast, broth thickened with rice, soft-cooked egg, cereal, fruit juice, gelatin, and custard may be given. The feedings should be small and should be given six times a day. As the patient improves, a more liberal diet may be given.

CORONARY OCCLUSION

Coronary occlusion occurs when one of the blood vessels of the heart becomes blocked, causing a myocardial infarction (MI) or heart attack. The patient must have absolute quiet and bed rest. For the first 3 or 4 days usually only fluids are allowed. Water and fruit juices may be given through the day, but the amount of fluids given must not exceed 1,500 ml., or approximately 1 1/2 quarts. On the fourth or fifth day, if the patient has shown improvement, he may be given a soft diet. Usually, to achieve cardiac rest, the diet is relatively low in calories (800 to 1,200) and should be moderately low in protein, low in fat, high in carbohydrate, and low in sodium. The patient must eat slowly and must chew his food well. The low-calorie diet brings not only some loss in body weight but also in reduction in basal metabolism and hence cardiac rest. After 4 to 6 weeks the number of calories may be raised to 1,500, or the individual's maintenance level, but the diet should continue to be moderately low in protein, low in fat, and high in carbohydrate.

ANGINA PECTORIS

Angina pectoris is characterized by pain around the heart and a sudden sharp pain radiating from the heart to the shoulder and down the left arm. The attacks may occur intermittently, but with proper rest and care the patient can recover. The diet should be such that it causes the least amount of work for the digestive organs.

The diet should be low in calories, especially if the patient is obese. The diet can be more liberal than the diet for the treatment of coronary occlusion. The food must be easily digested and divided into six small meals. The patient may have one cup of coffee a day if the physician permits.

CARDIAC FAILURE

There are two types of cardiac failure: compensated and decompensated. Any of the diseases discussed before can cause cardiac failure.

Compensated cardiac failure

In compensated cardiac failure, the heart is able to maintain adequate circulation to all parts of the body, usually by some enlargement of the heart and an increased pulse rate. The patient is usually able to perform his daily tasks by avoiding any hurry, undue excitement, or strenuous work.

Dietary treatment for compensated cardiac failure is as follows:

1. The patient must definitely reduce his weight if he is overweight and must adhere to a low-calorie diet even if he is not overweight.
2. Bulky meals must be avoided to prevent pressure on the heart.
3. Gas-forming vegetables should be avoided for the same reason.
4. Stimulants should be avoided or used sparingly.
5. Sodium must be restricted if edema is present.
6. The diet should be well-balanced, high in carbohydrate, moderately low in protein, and low in fat, with adequate vitamins and minerals
7. Fluids may be taken as desired.

Decompensated cardiac failure

In decompensated cardiac failure, congestive heart failure, the heart is unable to maintain adequate circulation to all parts of the body. The patient is short of breath because of the retarded flow of blood and because inadequate amounts of oxygen are carried to the lungs. Any exertion causes pain in the chest. As the disease progresses, edema usually develops.

Dietary treatment for decompensated cardiac failure is as follows:

1. Only water and fruit juices may be allowed at first, or the Karrell diet, which consists of 6 ounces of milk four times a day, may be given.
2. Later, as the patient improves, the following foods, without the addition of salt, may be added to the diet: cereal, milk toast, soft-cooked egg, gelatin, mashed or baked potato, pureed vegetables and fruits, custard, and plain puddings. Ice cream may also be given if it is eaten slowly. Small meals should be served six times a day to prevent the patient from becoming overtired at any one meal.

ATHEROSCLEROSIS

Atherosclerosis is a thickening of the walls of the blood vessels. It is often characterized by a rise in the blood cholesterol level and by an increase in the blood of lipoproteins, which are large molecules consisting of fat and protein.

The exact cause of atherosclerosis is not known. Most authorities agree that obesity and a sedentary life have some part in its development. The most debatable issue is the question of how much and what kind of fat intake is most effective in the prevention of artherosclerosis. It is true that in the United States in the past 30 or 35 years the dietary intake of fat has increased, physical activities have decreased, and tensions have increased. It has been stated that the unsaturated fats found in vegetable oils tend to lower the cholesterol and lipoprotein level of the blood if used in the diet in fairly large amounts. According to Dr. Ancel Keys of the University of Minnesota, about 2 ounces (4 tablespoons) of polyunsaturated fats will reduce the blood cholesterol level the same amount that 1 ounce (2 tablespoons) of saturated fat will increase it.

Lowering the intake of cholesterol in the diet does have some effect on the lowering of the blood cholesterol level although the body is able to manufacture cholesterol within itself. A low-saturated fat, low-cholesterol diet has also been effective in lowering the blood cholesterol level.

In view of all the findings, it is advisable to avoid overweight and to have a balanced diet that is low in animal fats and low in cholesterol. The diet should contain a moderate amount of protein from lean meats, poultry, and fish and a reasonable amount of fruits, vegetables, cereals, bread, and skimmed milk. Adequate vitamins and minerals should be given. If there is edema, sodium must be restricted. Fluids may be given as desired. The daily allowances of food on the low fat, low-cholesterol diet are as follows:

2 cups skimmed milk
6 oz. lean meat, poultry, or fish
1 serving cereal
6 slices bread

1 serving potatoes, rice, noodles, spaghetti, or macaroni
2 servings green or yellow vegetables
1 serving of another vegetable
3 servings fruit or fruit juice (1 a citrus fruit or fruit juice)

For additional calories use cereals, bread, fruits, vegetables, and skimmed milk. Since animal fats are omitted from the diet, it is evident that fat-soluble vitamins will be present only in limited amounts. The physician may wish to give a vitamin supplement.

For foods high in cholesterol, consult Table 4-1, which lists the cholesterol content of various types of foods.

HYPERTENSION

Hypertension is not a disease but a symptom of other conditions such as kidney disease, or it may be of unknown origin, so-called essential hypertension. Many times it is not discovered until a person has a routine physical examination. Sometimes he has headaches and dizziness and is short of breath. Many persons feel no ill effects from hypertension.

There is a thickening of the walls of the blood vessels that alters the flow of blood to the heart and kidneys and eventually damages these organs if the hypertension is severe. Although the blood pressure may decrease in some patients, there is no convincing evidence that the progress of the disease is retarded or arrested. The person with hypertension should develop a calm, unhurried, and unworried attitude toward life in general.

The dietary treatment for hypertension is as follows:

1. The patient should reduce his weight to normal or slightly below if he is obese or to 10% below his normal weight if he is not obese.
2. The energy value of the diet is limited to sufficient calories to maintain ideal body weight.
3. The protein should be the normal amount of 60 to 70 grams and of high biological value.
4. Approximately 50% of the calories should come from carbohydrates.
5. The diet should be moderately low in fats.
6. Adequate vitamins and minerals must be included in the diet.
7. Sodium should be restricted. Usually, with use of current anti-hypertensive drugs, only a mild restriction to about 2 grams of sodium daily is required.
8. Generous amounts of fruits and vegetables should be included in the diet.
9. Milk may also be included in the diet.

Questions on the cardiovascular system

1. Why is there a larger percentage of deaths from cardiovascular diseases today?
2. What are the objectives of the dietary treatment for heart patients?
3. What are the two types of cardiac disturbances? Describe each.
4. What changes in the heart occur in coronary occlusion?
5. Outline the dietary treatment for coronary occlusion.
6. How does angina pectoris manifest itself?
7. What type of diet should be given in the treatment of angina pectoris?
8. Name the two types of cardiac failure. Explain each.
9. List the modifications that should be made in the diet for a patient with compensated heart failure.
10. Outline the diet for a patient with decompensated heart failure.
11. What are the characteristic symptoms of atherosclerosis?
12. What are the probable causes of atherosclerosis?
13. Discuss the present theory in regard to the use of unsaturated fats.
14. What effect does lowering the dietary cholesterol have on the blood cholesterol?
15. What is the most effective diet to use in the treatment of atherosclerosis in the light of present-day knowledge?
16. Plan a low-fat, low-cholesterol diet for 2 days.
17. What are some of the characteristic symptoms of hypertension?
18. What occurs in the blood vessels in hypertension?
19. What are the specifications for the dietary treatment of hypertension? Discuss fully.

Suggestions for additional study

1. Plan a day's menu for a patient with hypertension.
2. Plan a day's menu for a patient with coronary occlusion for the first few days and another day's menu for the same patient 6 weeks later.

References

Christakis, G., and Winston, M.: Nutritional therapy in acute myocardial infarction, J. Am. Diet. Assoc. **63**:233, 1973.

Williams, S. R.: Nutrition and diet therapy, ed. 3, St. Louis, 1977, The C. V. Mosby Co.
Williams, S. R.: Essentials of nutrition and diet therapy, ed. 2, St. Louis, 1978, The C. V. Mosby Co.

21

Diabetes

Diabetes may be classified as a deficiency disease in which the ability to utilize glucose is impaired. This deficiency may be due to the failure of the pancreas to secrete sufficient insulin to take care of the glucose in a normal diet, or because the insulin produced is bound and unavailable for use. The normal pancreas supplies sufficient insulin to metabolize the carbohydrates in the body.

Sometimes a mild condition can be controlled by diet alone, but in the more severe conditions insulin is required. Insulin cannot be given by mouth, since it is a protein and would be digested; therefore, it must be given by injection.

At other times, oral hypoglycemic agents can be used effectively with some patients. The original oral drug product was given the name of Orinase; the chemical name is tolbutamide. Other oral hypoglycemics also used include chlorpropamide (Diabinese) and acetohexamide (Dymelor). A formerly used product, phenformin hydrochloride (DBI), has now been removed from the market.

The oral hypoglycemic agents are not effective in juvenile diabetes, and insulin must therefore be used. They are most effective in the milder cases of diabetes in adults over 35 years of age, and these patients must conform to the diet as much as if they were on insulin alone.

There are two types of diabetes. *Juvenile* diabetes is usually manifested before the age of 20 years. It is difficult to manage and requires both dietary restrictions and insulin for its control. Patients may experience wide fluctuations in blood sugar from day to day. *Adult* diabetes is usually developed after the age of 35 and is usually controlled by diet. Sometimes there may be a need for insulin. Adult-onset diabetes is usually milder in form than juvenile-onset diabetes.

An oral hypoglycemic agent may very well be used for older patients who cannot give themselves insulin as they should. It may also be used when insulin reactions must be avoided (as in a heart condition), when the patient is allergic to insulin, or when the patient refuses insulin.

The oral agents are not substitutes for insulin. Even though the patient takes an oral agent, there may be times of tension and strain when insulin would be better.

Although diabetes can be controlled, the cause of the disease is unknown and cannot be prevented. We do know that the disease is hereditary and that it has afflicted humans for centuries.

The diet of a diabetic person should be determined by his age, sex, body build, body weight, and degree of activity. The maintenance requirements are the same for a diabetic person as for a normal person.

The energy need of the person is based on sufficient calories to maintain ideal body weight. Usually for adults an allowance of about 30 calories per kilogram of ideal body weight is used. Approximately 1 gram of protein per kilogram body weight, or 20% of the total calories, is a baseline allowance.

The newly revised current recommendations for carbohydrate are liberalized to about 50% of the total calories, with the greater portion of this allowance (about 40%) in complex carbohydrates such as starch and the lesser portion (10%) for simple carbohydrates such as fruit. The new recommendation for fat is a moderate controlled amount, no more than 25% to 30% of the total calories, with limited use of animal fats.

Usually the exchange system of dietary control is used for planning the diabetic diet. The exchange system of dietary control, developed by professional organizations such as the American Dietetic Association, is based on a simple grouping of common foods according to generally equivalent nutritional values. This system may be used for any situation requiring calorie and food value control.

The foods are divided into six basic groups (some with subgroups), called the "exchange groups." Each food item within a group (or subgroup) contains approximately the same food value as any other food item in that group, allowing for exchange within groups and thus providing for variety in food choices as well as food value control. Hence the term "food exchanges" is used to refer to food choices or servings. The total number of exchanges per day depends upon individual nutritional needs, based on normal nutritional standards.

Suggested distributions of carbohydrate, protein, and fat for various amounts of calories are given in Table 21-1. These values reflect the new recommendations for nutrient ratios.

The meal plans given in Table 21-2 are only suggested meal plans. The individual food plan will allow for a patient's food preferences and economic status.

The principle of planning the diabetic diet by the simplified method is based on the plan of food exchanges. The common foods used are divided into six groups, as indicated in Table 21-4, according to their composition. The greatest advantage of the exchange system to the patient is that it gives the patient more freedom in selecting his food. The diet no longer needs to be monotonous, nor is the patient burdened by long lists of food values that are difficult for the average person to understand.

Table 21-1. Meal planning with exchange lists (American Dietetic Association)*

Diet	Calories	Carbo-hydrate (gm.) (50% of total calories)	Protein (gm.) (20% of total calories)	Fat (gm.) (30% of total calories)	Suggested carbohydrate distribution			
					Break-fast	Lunch	Dinner	Bed-time
1	1,200	150	60	40	25	50	50	25
2	1,500	185	75	50	32	62	62	30
3	1,800	225	90	60	38	75	75	37
4	2,200	275	110	75	46	92	92	46
5†	1,800	225	90	60	38	75	75	37
6†	2,600	325	130	85	54	108	108	54
7†	3,500	435	175	115	72	145	145	72
8	2,600	325	130	85	54	108	108	54
9	3,000	370	150	100	62	125	125	62

*Based on current recommendations for revised nutrient ratios and general distribution patterns by the American Diabetes Association, Inc., and the American Dietetic Association in cooperation with the Chronic Disease Program, United States Public Health Service, Department of Health, Education, and Welfare.
†These diets contain more milk and are especially su ble for children.

Table 21-2. Meal planning with exchange lists*

Diet	Milk‡	Vegetable A	Vegetable B	Fruits	Bread exchange	Meat exchange	Fat exchange
1	1 pt.	As desired	1	3	4	6	1
2	1 pt.	As desired	1	3	6	7	2
3	1 pt.	As desired	1	3	9	7	4
4	1 pt.	As desired	1	4	12	8	6
5†	1 qt.	As desired	1	3	7	6	3
6†	1 qt.	As desired	1	4	12	7	8
7†	1 qt.	As desired	1	6	20	10	10
8	1 pt.	As desired	1	4	15	10	10
9	1 pt.	As desired	1	4	17	10	12

*Based on current recommendations for revised nutrient ratios and general distribution patterns by committees of the American Diabetes Association, Inc., and the American Dietetic Association in cooperation with the Chronic Disease Program, United States Public Health Service, Department of Health, Education, and Welfare.
†These diets contain more milk and are especially suitable for children.
‡Lower fat milk (i.e., skim or low-fat) recommended.

Table 21-3. Food groups (exchanges) and their composition

Food	Approx. measure	Carbohydrate (gm.)	Protein (gm.)	Fat (gm.)	Calories
Milk exchanges	1 cup				
A (nonfat)		12	8	—	80
B (low-fat)		12	8	5	125
C (full-fat)		12	8	10	170
Vegetable exchanges					
A (low-carbohydrate)	as desired				Negligible
B (medium-carbohydrate)	1/2 cup	7	2	—	35
Fruit exchanges	Varies	10	—	—	40
Bread exchanges	1 slice	15	2	—	70
Meat exchanges	1 oz.				
A (lean)		—	7	3	55
B (medium-fat)		—	7	6	78
C (high-fat)		—	7	8	100
Fat exchanges	1 tsp.				
A (unsaturated)		—	—	5	45
B (monounsaturated)		—	—	5	45
C (saturated)		—	—	5	45

Table 21-4. Food exchange groups

List 1: Milk exchanges

(Cream portion of whole milk equals two fat exchanges. Hence, 1 cup whole milk equals 1 cup of skim milk plus two fat exchanges.)

Group A (nonfat)

Skim or nonfat milk	1 cup
Powdered, nonfat dry milk (before adding liquid)	1/3 cup
Canned, evaporated skim milk	1/2 cup
Buttermilk	1 cup
Yogurt made from skim milk (plain, unflavored)	1 cup

Group B (low-fat)

Low-fat milk (2% butterfat)	1 cup
Yogurt made from low-fat milk (plain, unflavored)	1 cup

Group C (full-fat)

Whole milk	1 cup
Canned, evaporated whole milk	1/2 cup
Powdered, whole dry milk (before adding liquid)	1/3 cup
Yogurt made from whole milk (plain, unflavored)	1 cup

List 2: Vegetable exchanges

(As served plain, without fat, seasoning, or dressing. Any fat used is taken from the fat exchange allowance.)

Group A (In amounts commonly eaten, use as desired.)

Asparagus	Broccoli	Celery
Bok choi, gai choi	Brussels sprouts	Chicory
Bamboo shoots	Cabbage	Chinese cabbage
Bean sprouts	Cauliflower	Cucumber

Table 21-4. Food exchange groups—cont'd

List 2: Vegetable exchanges—cont'd

Eggplant	Greens—cont'd	Rhubarb
Endive	mustard	Sauerkraut
Green pepper, chili pepper	spinach	Stringbeans: green, yellow, wax
Greens:	turnip	Summer squash
beet	Lettuce: all varieties	Tomatoes
chard	Mushrooms	Tomato juice
collards	Onions	Turnips
dandelion	Parsley	Vegetable juice, mixed
escarole	Pimientoes	Watercress
kale	Radishes	Zucchini

Group B (One serving equals $1/2$ cup unless otherwise stated.)

Artichoke (1 medium)	Green peas ($1/3$ cup)	Okra (8 or 9 pods)
Beets	Carrots (1 medium)	Rutabagas

List 3: Fruit exchanges
(Unsweetened: fresh, frozen, canned, cooked. One exchange is the portion indicated by the fruit.)

Berries		*Other fruits*	
Blackberries	$1/2$ cup	Apple	1 small
Blueberries	$1/2$ cup	Apple juice	$1/3$ cup
Raspberries	$1/2$ cup	Apple cider	$1/3$ cup
Strawberries	$3/4$ cup	Applesauce	$1/2$ cup
Citrus fruits		Apricots	2 medium
Grapefruit	$1/2$ small	Banana	$1/2$ small
Grapefruit juice	$1/2$ cup	Cherries	10 large, 17 small
Orange	1 small	Fig	1 large
Orange juice	$1/2$ cup	Fruit cocktail	$1/2$ cup
Tangerine	1 medium	Grapes	10 medium
Melons		Grape juice	$1/4$ cup
Canteloupe	$1/4$ medium	Kiwi fruit	1 medium
Honeydew	$1/8$ medium	Mango	$1/2$ small
Watermelon	1 cup, diced	Nectarine	1 small
(approx. $1/2$ center slice)		Papaya	$1/3$ medium, $1/2$ small
Dried fruits		Peach	1 medium
Apricots	4 halves	Pear	1 medium
Dates	2 medium	Persimmon	1 medium
Figs	1 medium	Pineapple	$1/2$ cup; 1 round
Prunes	2 medium		center slice
Peaches	2 halves	Pineapple juice	$1/3$ cup
Pears	2 halves	Plums	2 medium
Raisins	2 tbsp.	Prunes, fresh	2 medium
		Prune juice	$1/4$ cup

List 4: Bread exchanges
(Equivalent portions indicated by each item.)

Bread			
Bread (loaf, average size slice):	1 slice	Pumpernickel	1 slice
French		Raisin	
Italian		Rye	
White		Bagel	$1/2$
Whole wheat		English muffin	$1/2$

Continued.

Table 21-4. Food exchange groups—cont'd

List 4: Bread exchanges—cont'd

Bread—cont'd		Starchy vegetables	
Plain roll	1 small	Corn	1/3 cup
Frankfurter roll	1	Corn on cob (6-in. ear)	1/2 ear
Hamburger bun	1/2	Lima beans	1/2 cup
Dried bread crumbs	3 tbsp.	Parsnips	1/2 cup
Tortilla (6-in.)	1	Potato, white	1 small
Cereal		Potato, white mashed	1/2 cup
Dry cereal (ready-to-eat, unsweetened)		Pumpkin	1 cup
		Winter squash	1/2 cup
Bran flakes	1/2 cup	(acorn, butternut, banana)	
Grape Nuts	1/4 cup	Sweet potato	1/2 small;
Other (flake, puff)	3/4 cup		1/3 cup
Cereal, cooked	1/2 cup	Yam	1/2 small;
Bulgur, cooked	1/2 cup		1/3 cup
Grits, cooked	1/2 cup		
Pasta, cooked	1/2 cup	*Prepared foods*	
(spaghetti, noodles, macaroni)		Biscuit, 2″ diameter	1
Rice, cooked	1/2 cup	(omit 1 fat exchange)	
Popcorn (popped, no fat)	1 1/2 cup	Cornbread, 2″×2″×1 1/4″	1 square
Cornmeal, dry	2 tbsp.	(omit 1 fat exchange)	
Flour	2 1/2 tbsp.	Corn Muffin, 2″ diameter	1
Wheat germ, plain	3 tbsp.	(omit 1 fat exchange)	
Crackers		Crepes, 6″ diameter	1
Arrowroot	3	(omit 1 fat exchange)	
Graham, 2 1/2″ square	2	Muffin, plain, 2″ diameter	1
Matzoth, 4″ × 6″	1	(omit 1 fat exchange)	
Oyster crackers	20	Potatoes, French fried	8 pieces
Pretzels, 3 1/8″ × 1/8″	25	(length 2-3″; omit 1 fat)	
Round, butter-type crackers	6	Chips, potato or corn	15
Rye wafers, 2″ × 3 1/2″	3	(omit 2 fat exchanges)	
Saltines	5	Pancakes, 4″ diameter	1
Soda crackers, 2 1/2″ square	3	(omit 1 fat exchange)	
Dried beans, peas, lentils		Waffle, 4″ diameter or square	1
Beans, peas, lentils	1/3 cup	(omit 1 fat exchange)	
(dried and cooked)		Ice milk, 1/2 cup scoop	1 scoop
Baked beans, no pork	1/4 cup	(omit 1 fat exchange)	
		Angel food cake	1 slice
		(1 1/2″ cube or small slice)	
		Sherbet, fruit ice, 1/2 cup scoop	1 scoop

List 5: Meat exchanges

(Lean meat, trimmed well)

Group A (Lean; low in saturated fat and cholesterol)

   I. *Lean meats, less tissue fat*

Fish: Any fresh or frozen	1 oz.	Poultry (no skin)	1 oz
Canned salmon, tuna, mackerel	1/4 cup	Chicken, turkey, cornish hen, guinea hen, pheasant	
Sardines, drained	3	Veal: Any lean, trimmed	1 oz
Shellfish			
Crab, lobster	1/4 cup		
Clams, oysters, scallops	5		

Table 21-4. Food exchange groups—cont'd

List 5: Meat exchanges—cont'd

II. *Lean meats, more tissue fat*

Beef	1 oz.	Lamb	1 oz.
Very lean young beef; chipped beef; lean cuts: chuck, flank steak, tenderloin, plate ribs and skirt steak, round (top, bottom), rump, spare ribs, tripe		Lean cuts: leg, rib sirloin, loin (roast, chops), shank, shoulder	
		Pork	1 oz
		Lean cuts: leg (rump, center shank), ham (smoked center cut)	

III. *Cheese*

Cottage cheese $1/4$ cup
    Dry curd
    Low-fat partially recreamed
Other cheeses   1 oz.
    Less than 5% butterfat;
    partially skim milk

Group B (Medium-fat)

Beef	1 oz	Cholesterol foods	
Ground (15% fat)		Organ meats:	1 oz.
Corned (canned)		Liver, kidney, sweetbreads	
Pork	1 oz.	Heart	1 oz.
Loin (roast, chops), shoulder, arm (picnic), shoulder blade, Boston butt, Canadian bacon, boiled ham		Egg	1
		Shrimp	5 large
		Other:	
Cheese	1 oz.	Peanut butter	2 tbsp.
Mozzarella, ricotta, swiss, jack, farmer's, neufachtel		(omit 2 fat exchanges)	
Parmesan	3 tbsp.	Tofu	$3^1/2$ oz.
Cottage	$1/4$ cup		

Group C (High-fat)

Beef	1 oz.	Cold cuts	1 slice
Brisket (fresh or corned)		Frankfurter	1 small
Ground (20% or more fat)		Cheese, cheddar types	1 oz.
Lamb	1 oz.	Poultry	1 oz.
Breast		Capon, duck, goose	
Pork	1 oz.		
Spareribs, back ribs, ground pork, sausage, country style ham, deviled ham			

List 6: Fat exchanges

Group A (Polyunsaturated plant fats)

Margarine* soft (stick or tub)	1 tsp.
Mocha mix (cream substitute)	2 tbsp.
Nuts: Walnuts	4-5 halves
Vegetable oils	1 tsp.
Safflower, corn, soy, cottonseed, sesame	
Salad dressings *	
French	1 tbsp.
Italian	1 tbsp.
Mayonnaise	1 tsp.
Seeds (sunflower, sesame, pumpkin)	1 tbsp.

*Made with safflower, corn, soy, cottonseed oil.

Continued.

Table 21-4. Food exchange groups—cont'd

List 6: Fat exchanges—cont'd

Group B (monounsaturated plant fats)	
Avocado	$1/_8$
Nuts	
Almonds	10 whole
Peanuts	20 whole
Pecans	2 whole
Olives	5 small
Vegetable oils	1 tsp.
Olive, peanut	
Group C (saturated animal fats)	
Butter	1 tsp.
Cheese spreads	1 tbsp.
Cream	
Half & half (10% cream)	2 tbsp.
Light (20% cream)	2 tbsp.
Heavy (40% cream)	1 tbsp.
Sour (light)	2 tbsp.
Cream cheese	1 tbsp.
Pork fat	
Bacon, crisp	1 strip
Bacon fat	1 tsp.
Lard	1 tsp.
Salt pork	$3/_4$ in. cube

Miscellaneous foods allowed as desired
(Negligible carbohydrate, protein, fat)

Artificial sweeteners, as permitted	Gelatin, plain, or D-Zerta
Bouillon, broth, clear fat-free	Herbs and spices
Catsup, mustard, horseradish, meat sauce	Lemon, lime
Coffee, tea	Pickles, dill and sour
Cranberries, cranberry juice (unsweetened)	Salt and pepper
Garlic	Vinegar

Table 21-3 lists the new, revised food exchange groups and their composition. Although there is some variation in the composition of foods within the exchange groups, for simplicity the values given in the table for carbohydrate, protein, fat, and calories are used for general calculations.

Table 21-4 gives new, revised food exchange lists, incorporating the greater attention being given to control of fat, especially saturated (animal) fat.

The chart on p. 153 may be used in planning daily menus for a diabetic person.

"Specialty" foods for diabetic patients are unnecessary. They are expensive, and the information on the package can be misleading. They are not needed, for diabetic persons can usually eat all the natural primary foods (breads, cereals, unsweetened fruits, vegetables, and so forth) in the proper amounts.

Meal plan	Foods	Household measures	Grams
Breakfast _____ Fruit exchange _____ Bread exchange _____ Meat exchange _____ Milk exchange _____ Fat exchange			
Lunch _____ Meat exchange _____ Bread exchange _____ Vegetable–Group A _____ Vegetable–Group B _____ Fruit exchange _____ Milk exchange _____ Fat exchange			
Dinner _____ Meat exchange _____ Bread exchange _____ Vegetable–Group A _____ Vegetable–Group B _____ Fruit exchange _____ Milk exchange _____ Fat exchange			
Bedtime			

Questions on diabetes

1. What is diabetes?
2. Why is insulin usually necessary?
3. Why cannot insulin be taken by mouth?
4. For what type of patient is the oral hypoglycemic agent the most effective?
5. Is dietary control necessary when the oral agent is used?
6. How many calories per pound should be allowed for the diabetic patient? How many grams of protein should be allowed?
7. Why do some physicians prescribe larger amounts of protein?
8. What is the most frequently prescribed ratio of carbohydrate, protein, and fat?
9. What are the advantages of using the exchange system?
10. Name the six groups of foods used in the exchange system.
11. Why are "specialty" foods for diabetic persons not recommended?
12. Name two foods in each exchange list.
13. How many calories are in each of the six exchange groups?
14. Name two substitutes for each of the following: 1 slice bread, 1/2 cup orange juice, 1 tsp. butter, 1 egg.
15. List six of the "free" foods (Table 21-4).
16. Plan a 1,200-calorie diabetic diet based on the American Dietetic Association's sample meal plan (diet 1).

Suggestions for additional study

1. A patient on a diabetic diet receives chicken and asparagus and will not eat either one. What can be substituted?
2. Make substitutions for the following on a diabetic diet, listing the quantities: 4 apricot halves, 2 graham crackers, $1^1/_2$-inch cube sponge cake, 3 oz. roast beef, 1 strip bacon, 1 slice bread, 2 prunes, tossed salad, 1 glass whole milk, $^1/_2$ cup beets.

References

American Dietetic Association: Meal planning with exchange lists, rev. ed., Chicago, 1977, The Association.

Williams, S. R.: Nutrition and diet therapy, ed. 3, St. Louis, 1977, The C. V. Mosby Co.

Williams, S. R.: Essentials of nutrition and diet therapy, ed. 2, St. Louis, 1978, The C. V. Mosby Co.

22

Obesity

Overweight is one of the most common medical problems today. It is estimated that approximately 5 million Americans weight at least 20% more than their normal weight. Another 20 million are classified by physicians as being 10% above normal in weight.

In the past, a fat person was thought of as a healthy person. This was especially true in regard to babies. The present desire to avoid overweight has come into prominence largely for two reasons: the slender figure is more fashionable, and data based on scientific studies show that life expectancy is influenced to a considerable extent by body weight.

Obesity may be defined as an abnormal condition due to excessive deposits of fat in the body that result in overweight. Obesity from glandular abnormality is very rare. A tendency toward overweight and certain factors that increase hunger may be inherited, but the fat itself is not. The cause of overweight in most cases is simply eating too much. Overweight places an added burden on the heart, circulatory system, liver, and gallbladder. It also increases the risk in surgery and hypertension. It is thought to be a predisposing factor in diabetes, gout, and arthritis. Most overweight people have trouble with their feet. The bones of the feet were meant to carry only a certain amount of weight, and when this is greatly increased, trouble results.

Since overweight is for the most part the result of overeating, what, then, are the causes of overeating? A person who is bored or unhappy is more likely to snack between meals than a well-adjusted person. Some persons have a family history of members who consistently overate and who made no effort to limit the amount consumed. Children are sometimes rewarded for good behavior with tempting bits of food; therefore, they associate obedience with overeating. A person with a psychological problem may overeat to gain a temporary sense of well-being.

An effort to avoid obesity has both good and bad results. In many cases it has led to a better selection of food. However, there are people who harm themselves by trying to reduce unwisely. It is very important that a person trying to

reduce receive the necessary protein, minerals, and vitamins for adequate nutrition.

The so-called fad diets for reducing should be discouraged. In the first
place, many of them are inadequate; in the second place, they do nothing to
educate the person in good eating habits. This is important because often a person who has lost weight on a fad diet will resume his former eating habits after
losing weight and will soon be right back where he started.

A good reducing diet should lay the foundation for a sensible diet regimen
that can, with some additions, be followed indefinitely. Once the loss in weight
has been achieved, a person may gradually add more foods, checking his weight
at least once a week. If he begins to gain weight, he should return at once to his
former reducing regimen.

Most authorities advocate that a person's ideal weight at 25 years of age is
the best weight to maintain for the rest of his life. If this is to be accomplished,
calories must be reduced 3% from 30 to 40 years of age, another 3% from 40 to
50 years of age, 7.5% from 50 to 60 years of age, and another 7.5% from 60 to 70
years of age. In fact, the term "middle-aged spread" is a misnomer. There is no
mysterious law of nature that states that all persons must enlarge horizontally at
middle age. An excessive increase in weight at this time of life is simply the result of too many calories and too little exercise. A person's normal body weight
is determined not only by age but also by height and body build. For example,
a person with large bones can carry more weight without being obese than a
person with small bones.

A certain amount of moderate exercise is good to maintain physical well-
being. People who are physically active are less likely to be overweight. Exercise, however, cannot take the place of diet. Regular exercise, especially for
younger people, makes flabby muscles firmer and helps to achieve more attractive proportions. Even middle-aged persons who are on reducing diets should
plan some sort of moderate, consistent exercise program.

The use of drugs to help a person reduce should be discouraged, and is not
advocated by any reputable physician now. Some produce extremely toxic effects, and some have a harmful cumulative effect that may not be felt for some
time. Thyroid preparations are sometimes given, but unless the thyroid gland is
actually deficient, they should never be taken.

The best and safest plan for reducing is, as it has always been, to lower the
calorie intake below the actual daily needs of the body, making it necessary for
the body to draw upon and use its reserve fat.

The reduction in food must come primarily from carbohydrates and fats.
Protein is necessary at all times for the repair of body tissues and should be
maintained at a higher than normal level. Protein foods such as meat, eggs, fish,
and cottage cheese have a high satiety value. A patient on a reducing diet will
be better satisfied and better nourished on a high-protein, low-carbohydrate,
low-fat diet. Low-calorie vegetables and fruits will add interest to the diet and

furnish needed vitamins, minerals, and bulk. The essentials of a reducing diet, then, include the following:

1. There should be sufficient high-quality protein to prevent wasting of body tissues and to furnish adequate protein for body processes.
2. There should be sufficient carbohydrate to prevent protein from being used for energy needs and to prevent too rapid burning of body fat.
3. Adequate minerals and vitamins must be provided.
4. The diet should be acceptable to the patient.
5. The diet should be one that will educate the patient in correct eating habits.
6. Meals should not be skipped.

An adequate breakfast gives the person a proper start for the day. There should be some protein food in each meal, especially breakfast. Carbohydrate alone raises the blood sugar quickly but not for long, whereas protein raises the blood sugar level and holds it above the hunger mark longer.

The caloric value of the diet may be cut safely to 1,200 calories. Below 1,200 calories, a diet is not adequate, and a person on such a diet should have very close nutritional supervision.

An adult who is overweight has probably been consuming at least 3,000 calories daily and often more than that amount. In a reducing diet, the caloric reduction should start from a person's ideal caloric allowance and not from the number of calories he has been consuming. For the person whose ideal caloric intake is 2,200, a cut of 1,000 calories should result in a weight loss of approximately 2 pounds a week, and a daily reduction of 500 calories from the person's ideal caloric intake will, under normal conditions, result in a weight loss of 1 pound per week.

EXAMPLE: A woman 35 years of age weighs 148 pounds, but her ideal weight is 125 pounds.

2,200 calories needed to maintain person at 125 pounds
−1,000
1,200 calorie diet necessary to lose an average of 2 pounds a week

It should take the patient 10 weeks to lose the 20 pounds. There may be a variation in the weekly loss of weight, depending upon the activity of the patient, variations in the water balance of the body, and the presence of disease.

The person who is on a reducing diet may plan to weigh himself about once a week. Otherwise, he becomes discouraged when each day does not show a loss. At first the fat in the tissues may be replaced by water, and the person may not show a loss. It took time to put on the extra pounds, and it will take time to lose them.

Dieting can bring rewards when it is well planned, using a variety of foods. Instead of reaching for a rich dessert, one may choose fresh fruit. After the first few days it becomes easier. If one diets sensibly, he will not be hungry or

Table 22-1. Desirable weights for men 25 years of age and over (in indoor clothing)*

Height (with shoes on) 1-inch heels		Small frame	Medium frame	Large frame
Feet	Inches			
5	2	112-120	118-129	126-141
5	3	115-123	121-133	129-144
5	4	118-126	124-136	132-148
5	5	121-129	127-139	135-152
5	6	124-133	130-143	138-156
5	7	128-137	134-147	142-161
5	8	132-141	138-152	147-166
5	9	136-145	142-156	151-170
5	10	140-150	146-160	155-174
5	11	144-154	150-165	159-179
6	0	148-158	154-170	164-184
6	1	152-162	158-175	168-189
6	2	156-167	162-180	173-194
6	3	160-171	167-185	178-199
6	4	164-175	172-190	182-204

*Courtesy Metropolitan Life Insurance Co., New York, N.Y.

Table 22-2. Desirable weights for women 25 years of age and over (in indoor clothing)*

Height (with shoes on) 2-inch heels		Small frame	Medium frame	Large frame
Feet	Inches			
4	10	92-98	96-107	104-119
4	11	94-101	98-110	106-122
5	0	96-104	101-113	109-125
5	1	99-107	104-116	112-128
5	2	102-110	107-119	115-131
5	3	105-113	110-122	118-134
5	4	108-116	113-126	121-138
5	5	111-119	116-130	125-142
5	6	114-123	120-135	129-146
5	7	118-127	124-139	133-150
5	8	122-131	128-143	137-154
5	9	126-135	132-147	141-158
5	10	130-140	136-151	145-163
5	11	134-144	140-155	149-168
6	0	138-148	144-159	153-173

*Courtesy Metropolitan Life Insurance Co., New York, N.Y.
For girls between 18 and 25 years of age, subtract 1 lb. for each year under 25.

tempted too strongly to choose the higher-calorie foods. He should not over-step the diet. The stomach is an indisputable adding machine. Alcoholic beverages are very high in calories and should be avoided in a reducing diet. Weight reduction food plans can use the same food exchange system presented in the preceding chapter for diabetes control (Tables 21-3 and 21-4).

Daily diet patterns for reduction diets

1,500-calorie diet

1 fruit exchange (unsweetened)
2 fruit exchanges (lightly sweetened)
1 vegetable B exchange
3 vegetable A exchanges
3 bread exchanges
7 meat exchanges
3 fat exchanges
1 pt. whole milk
2 tsp. sugar

CARBOHYDRATE	145
PROTEIN	70
FAT	70

1,200 calories

3 fruit exchanges

1 vegetable B exchange
3 vegetable A exchanges
3 bread exchanges
7 meat exchanges
2 fat exchanges
1 pt. skim milk

CARBOHYDRATE	115
PROTEIN	75
FAT	45

1,000 calories

3 fruit exchanges
1 vegetable B exchange
3 vegetable A exchanges
1 bread exchange
7 meat exchanges
1 fat exchange
1 pt. skim milk

CARBOHYDRATE	85
PROTEIN	70
FAT	40

800 calories

3 fruit exchanges
1 vegetable B exchange
3 vegetable A exchanges
1 bread exchange
6 meat exchanges

1 cup skim milk

CARBOHYDRATE	75
PROTEIN	55
FAT	30

SAMPLE MENUS

Breakfast	Lunch	Dinner
1,500 calories		
¹/₂ grapefruit	Clear broth	Clear broth
Poached egg	3 oz. hamburger steak	3 oz. roast leg of lamb
1 slice whole-wheat bread, toasted	Fresh spinach	¹/₂ cup peas
	Tomato salad	Tossed salad
1 tsp. butter	1 slice bread	1 slice bread
2 tsp. sugar	1 tsp. butter	1 tsp. butter
1 cup homogenized milk	4 canned apricot halves (in light syrup)	10 Royal Anne cherries (in light syrup)
Coffee	Tea	1 cup whole milk

Breakfast	Lunch	Dinner

1,200 calories

$^1/_2$ grapefruit	Clear broth	Clear broth
Poached egg	3 oz. hamburger steak	3 oz. roast leg of lamb
1 slice bread, toasted	Fresh spinach	$^1/_2$ cup peas
1 tsp. butter	Tomato salad	Tossed salad
Coffee	1 slice bread	1 slice bread
	$^1/_2$ tsp. butter	$^1/_2$ tsp. butter
	4 canned apricot halves	10 Royal Anne cherries
	1 cup skim milk	1 cup skim milk

1,000 calories

$^1/_2$ grapefruit	3 oz. hamburger steak	Clear broth
Poached egg	Fresh spinach	3 oz. roast leg of lamb
1 slice bread, toasted	Tomato salad	$^1/_2$ cup peas
1 tsp. butter	4 canned apricot halves	Tossed salad
Coffee	1 cup skim milk	10 Royal Anne cherries
		1 cup skim milk

800 calories

$^1/_2$ grapefruit	Clear broth	Clear broth
Poached egg	2 oz. hamburger steak	3 oz. roast leg of lamb
1 slice bread, toasted	Fresh spinach	$^1/_2$ cup peas
Coffee	Tomato salad	Tossed salad
	4 canned apricot halves	10 Royal Anne cherries
	Tea	1 cup skim milk

1,500 calorie diet
(Carbohydrate, 142 grams; protein, 75 grams; fat, 70 grams)

Breakfast
   Choice of (40 calories): 1 serving cantaloupe, $^1/_4$ 6-in. diam. melon; grapefruit, $^1/_2$
      small; grapefruit juice, $^1/_2$ cup; orange, 1 small; orange juice, $^1/_2$ cup; pineapple
      juice, $^1/_3$ cup; tomato juice, 1 cup
   Egg (75 calories): 1 poached, soft-cooked, hard-cooked, or scrambled without addi-
      tion of any milk or butter other than that allowed in diet
   Toast (70 calories): 1 slice, whole-wheat or enriched preferred
      OR
   Cereal, $^1/_2$ cup cooked cereal or $^3/_4$ cup dry cereal
   Butter (45 calories): 1 tsp.
   Milk (170 calories): 1 cup whole milk
   Sugar (40 calories): 2 tsp.
   Coffee or tea as desired
Lunch
   Clear broth without any fat (no calories)
   Choice of (225 calories): 3 oz. lean beef, veal, lamb, fowl, or fish (all meat broiled,
      boiled, or roasted)
      OR

Cottage cheese: ³/₄ cup
> OR

American cheese: 3 thin slices
> OR

Egg: 1 poached, soft-cooked, hard-cooked, or scrambled, *and* ¹/₂ cup cottage cheese

Vegetables, choice of (15 calories each serving): 2 medium servings asparagus, broccoli, Brussels sprouts, cabbage, cauliflower, celery, cucumbers, eggplant, string beans, kale, lettuce, mushrooms, okra, radishes, sauerkraut, spinach, summer squash, or tomatoes

Bread (70 calories): 1 slice, whole-wheat or enriched preferred
> OR

Potato: 1 small
> OR

Rice, spaghetti, or noodles: ¹/₂ cup cooked

Butter (45 calories): 1 tsp.

Dessert: Choice of any of following fruits canned in light syrup (80 calories), applesauce, ¹/₂ cup; apricots, canned, 4 halves; blackberries, 1 cup; cherries, red or white, 10; fruit cocktail, ¹/₂ cup; gooseberries, 1 cup; peach, 2 halves; pear, 2 halves; raspberries, 1 cup; pineapple, ¹/₂ cup; plums, 2
> OR

Choice of any of following fresh fruits without any sugar added (40 calories): apple, 1 small; apricots, 2; blackberries, 1 cup; cherries, 10; cranberries, ¹/₂ cup; gooseberries, 1 cup; grapes, American, 12; grapes, green seedless, 33; grapes, Tokay, 12; peach, 1 small; pear, 1 small; raspberries, 1 cup; strawberries, 1 cup; pineapple, ¹/₂ cup; plums, 2 medium; watermelon, 1 cup.

Coffee or tea as desired (no sugar)

Dinner

Clear broth (no calories)

Choice of (225 calories): 3 oz. lean beef, veal, lamb, fowl, or fish (all meat broiled, boiled, or roasted)
> OR

Cottage cheese: ³/₄ cup
> OR

American cheese: 3 thin slices
> OR

Egg. 1 poached, soft-cooked, hard-cooked, or scrambled *and* ¹/₂ cup cottage cheese

Choice of (35 calories): ¹/₂ cup beets, carrots, onions, peas, or winter squash

Choice of (15 calories): 1 medium serving asparagus, broccoli, Brussels sprouts, cabbage, cauliflower, celery, cucumber, eggplant, string beans, kale, lettuce, mushrooms, okra, radishes, sauerkraut, spinach, summer squash, or tomatoes

Bread (70 calories): 1 slice, whole-wheat or enriched preferred
> OR

Potato: 1 small
> OR

Rice, spaghetti, or noodles: ¹/₂ cup cooked

Butter (45 calories): 1 tsp.

Dessert: Choice as at noon, or custard made with a sugar substitute (if custard used, omit 1 oz. meat and ¹/₂ cup milk and use fruit as salad or bedtime snack)
> OR

$^1/_2$ cup ice cream may be substituted occasionally for 1 cup whole milk

Milk (170 calories): 1 cup whole milk

1,200 calorie diet
(Carbohydrate, 114 grams; protein, 75 grams; fat, 45 grams)

Breakfast

Choice of (40 calories):1 serving cantaloupe, $^1/_4$ 6 in. diam. melon; grapefruit, $^1/_2$ small; grapefruit juice, $^1/_2$ cup; orange, 1 small; orange juice, $^1/_2$ cup; pineapple juice, $^1/_3$ cup; tomato juice, 1 cup

Egg (75 calories): 1 poached, soft-cooked, hard-cooked, or scrambled without addition of any milk or butter other than that allowed in diet

Toast (70 calories): 1 slice, whole-wheat or enriched preferred

Butter (45 calories): 1 tsp.

Coffee or tea as desired

Lunch

Clear broth without any fat (no calories)

Choice of (225 calories): 3 oz. lean beef, veal, lamb, fowl, or fish (all meat broiled, boiled, or roasted)

OR

Cottage cheese: $^3/_4$ cup

OR

American cheese: 3 thin slices

OR

Egg: 1 poached, soft-cooked, hard-cooked or scrambled *and* $^1/_2$ cup cottage cheese

Choice of (15 calories each serving): 2 medium servings asparagus, broccoli, Brussels sprouts, cabbage, cauliflower, celery, cucumbers, eggplant, string beans, kale, lettuce, mushrooms, okra, radishes, sauerkraut, spinach, summer squash, or tomatoes

Bread (70 calories): 1 slice, whole-wheat or enriched preferred

Butter (22 calories): $^1/_2$ tsp.

Dessert (40 calories): Choice of apple, 1 small; applesauce, $^1/_2$ cup; apricot, canned, 4 halves; apricots, fresh, 2; blackberries, 1 cup; cherries, red or white, 10; cranberries, fresh, $^1/_2$ cup (may be sweetened with saccharin and used as sauce for meat); fruit cocktail, $^1/_2$ cup; gooseberries, fresh, 1 cup; grapes, American, 12; grapes, green seedless, 33; grapes, Tokay, 12; peach, fresh, 1 small; peach, canned, 2 halves; pear, fresh, 1 small; pear, canned, 2 halves; raspberries, canned, 1 cup; strawberries, fresh, 1 cup; pineapple, fresh, $^1/_2$ cup; pineapple, canned, $^1/_2$ cup; plums, fresh, 2, medium; or watermelon, 1 cup

Milk: 1 cup skim milk or buttermilk

Coffee or tea as desired (no sugar)

Dinner

Clear broth (no calories)

Choice of (225 calories): 3 oz. lean beef, veal, lamb, fowl or fish (all meat broiled, boiled, or roasted)

OR

Cottage cheese: $^3/_4$ cup

OR

American cheese: 3 thin slices

OR

Egg: 1 poached, soft-cooked, hard-cooked, or scrambled *and* ¹/₂ cup cottage cheese

Choice of (35 calories): ¹/₂ cup beets, carrots, onions, peas, winter squash, or turnips

Choice of (15 calories each serving): 1 medium serving asparagus, broccoli, Brussels sprouts, cabbage, cauliflower, celery, cucumber, eggplant, string beans, kale, lettuce, mushrooms, okra, radishes, sauerkraut, spinach, summer squash, or tomatoes

Bread (70 calories): 1 slice, whole-wheat or enriched bread preferred

OR

Potato: 1 small

Butter (22 calories): ¹/₂ tsp.

Dessert: Choice as at noon, or custard made with a sugar substitute (if custard used, omit 1 oz. meat and ¹/₂ cup milk; use allowed fruit as a salad or as bedtime snack)

Milk: 1 cup skim milk or buttermilk

1,000 calorie diet and 800 calorie diet

Use the same general meal plan, following the daily diet patterns for 800 and 1,000 calorie diets given in this chapter.

The following general dietary rules apply to all the diets given above:

1. Vinegar, lemon juice, or a slice of lemon may be used on vegetables or salads. Mayonnaise or oil dressing should not be used.
2. Fat, cream, butter, or flour should not be used in the preparation of food.
3. A sugar substitute in moderation may be used instead of sugar.
4. Artificially sweetened or unsweetened gelatin may be used in making salads and desserts.
5. Fruit should never have sugar added. They may be eaten raw or cooked. Only water-packed canned fruit, except on the 1,500 calorie diet, may be used.

Questions on obesity

1. Why is overweight a health hazard?
2. What are some of the causes of overeating?
3. What are the characteristics of a good reducing diet?
4. Why should drugs not be used for reducing purposes?
5. What is the lowest caloric intake that will give an adequate diet?
6. What should the caloric reduction be for an approximate weight loss of 2 pounds a week?
7. Plan a 1,200-calorie diet and a 1,000-calorie diet for 3 days.

Suggestions for additional study

1. A person whose normal weight should be 135 pounds but who weighs 155 pounds wants to lose approximately 2 pounds a week. What should be the normal caloric intake if the ideal weight is 135 pounds, and what should be the caloric intake on a reduction diet?
2. Make a list of products that are commonly used to decrease the appetite.

3. Plan a minimum caloric diet that will meet the basic nutritional requirements.
4. Circle the correct answers in the right column to answer the questions in the left column.

Does obesity increase the load on the heart?	Yes No
Is a breakfast of sweet roll and black coffee adequate nutritionally?	Yes No
Is the cause of overweight overactive glands in most persons?	Yes No
Is chocolate cake a wise choice on a 1,000-calorie diet? Give the reason for your answer.	Yes No

References

Mayer, J.: Overweight, Englewood Cliffs, N.J., 1968, Prentice-Hall, Inc.

Stuart, R. B., and Davis, B.:. Slim chance in a fat world, Champaign, Ill., 1972, Research Press.

Williams, S. R.: Nutrition and diet therapy, ed. 3, St. Louis, 1977, The C. V. Mosby Co., Chapter 24.

Williams, S. R.: Essentials of nutrition and diet therapy, ed. 2, St. Louis, 1978, The C. V. Mosby Co.

23

Underweight

Extremes in underweight, just as in overweight, tend to shorten an individual's life-span. Although underweight is a much less common problem than overweight, it does occur. It is often more difficult to reach the underlying cause and the subsequent cure in the underweight person than in the overweight person.

A person who is more than 10% below the normal weight is considered to be underweight. Twenty percent or more below normal weight is cause for concern because serious results may occur, especially in persons in younger age groups. Resistance to infection is lowered, general health is below par, and efficiency is reduced.

Some of the causes of underweight are as follows:
1. Long, wasting disease with chronic elevated temperature that raises the basal metabolism
2. Diminished food intake due to (a) psychological reasons that cause a patient to refuse to eat, (b) anorexia or complete loss of appetite, or (c) economic reasons that curtail available food supply
3. Diminished food absorption due to (a) diarrhea of long duration, (b) an abnormal condition in the gastrointestinal tract, or (c) the excessive use of laxatives
4. Hyperthyroidism or any other abnormality that would increase the caloric needs of the body
5. Greatly increased activity without a corresponding increase in food
6. Unhealthy home environment, with irregular and inadequate meals, in which eating is considered unimportant and in which an indifferent attitude toward food is fostered

The purpose of a special diet for the person who is underweight is to provide a sufficiently high caloric intake so that he will gain the required amount of weight and at the same time establish good food habits. Unless good food habits are formed, a person will slip back into the former way of eating, and the problem will repeat itself.

The dietary requirements in the treatment of underweight result in the following type of diet:

1. High in calories, at least 50% above the person's normal requirement
2. High in protein since there has probably been some loss of body protein
3. High in carbohydrates since they are easily digested
4. Normal or a little below normal in fat since foods too high in fat are sometimes not very well tolerated
5. Normal amounts of minerals, except calcium and iron, which should be increased
6. High in vitamins, especially thiamine, which should be increased with an increase in carbohydrates (thiamine should stimulate the appetite)
7. Adequate in all the nutrients
8. Well-prepared and attractively served food to tempt the person with a poor appetite

There should be three meals daily, with high caloric nourishment between meals and in the evening. Rest before and after meals is beneficial. Because an underweight person often has little or no appetite, it is especially important that he be served the foods he likes.

The additional calories should be added to the diet gradually since the sudden change from a reduced intake to a 3,000- or 4,000-calorie intake may upset the patient. Bulky, low-calorie foods should be kept to a minimum if the patient is having difficulty in consuming all of his food.

Moderate exercise, such as walking, should be taken when possible to stimulate the appetite, to maintain general health, and to improve muscle tone.

The development of good food habits and a proper gain in weight should be the determining factors in measuring the success of the treatment of the patient who is underweight.

Questions on underweight

1. What percentage below normal is considered underweight?
2. What are the results of underweight?
3. What are some of the causes of underweight?
4. Plan a diet for an underweight person.

Reference

Robinson, C. H.: Basic nutrition and diet therapy, ed. 2, N.Y., 1970, The Macmillan Co., pp. 225-226.

24

Allergy

Allergy is a condition produced by allergens. An allergen is any substance to which a person is hypersensitive. Allergy may manifest itself as asthma, eczema, hives, swelling of the eyes, headache, or gastrointestinal ailments. The same effect may appear in different persons but still not be caused by the same allergen. Allergens enter the body in four different ways: by being swallowed (food and drinks), by being inhaled (pollen, animal dander, and dust), by external contact (clothing, cosmetics, and poisonous plants), and by injection (drugs, serums, and insect stings).

Although not all allergic manifestations are caused by a hypersensitivity to food, only this phase of allergy is discussed in this chapter.

Sometimes a person can eat food to which he is allergic without any ill effects, whereas at other times they affect him, Sometimes, when a person is allergic to more than one item, he can tolerate one of them at a time without incurring any unfortunate results. Tests for allergy should be taken twice since an allergy may not show up the first time.

The foods that most often cause allergic conditions are wheat, milk, eggs, tomatoes strawberries, oranges, fish, chocolate, nuts, peas, beans, potatoes, onions, and garlic. In asthma, wheat, and eggs are likely to head the list of causative allergens. In headache, wheat and chocolate may be guilty. Cooked vegetables are frequently tolerated by people who are allergic to raw ones. Many people are allergic to only the peel of peaches and can eat the peach if the peel is removed.

Fatigue, nervousness, tension, unhappiness, indigestion, or certain phases of the menstrual cycle may lower the tolerance and make a person more susceptible to an allergen.

Heredity is a factor in the appearance of an allergy. The evidence of an allergy in the child may appear in a different locale in the body from that in the adult from whom he inherited the tendency. His allergy may even be caused by a different substance from that caused by the adult's allergy.

Children seem to develop allergies more readily than adults. It usually attacks children in the form of eczema or asthma, and unless the allergy is kept under control, the condition may grow worse as the child grows older. Food is usually the source of allergies in very young children. The foods to which children are most often allergic are wheat, eggs, and milk. If a child is allergic to whole milk, it is usually possible for him to take milk in some other form, such as boiled milk, dry skim milk, or evaporated milk, or he may be able to tolerate goat's milk or soybean milk. Heating milk reduces the allergenic effect of lactalbumin, the milk protein fraction usually responsible for milk allergy. Children usually outgrow an allergy to milk.

The offending item may be determined by an elimination diet or, if one par-

Table 24-1. Elimination diets*

Diet 1	Diet 2	Diet 3	Diet 4
Rice	Corn	Tapioca	Milk, up to 2 to 3 qt. daily
Tapioca	Rye	White and sweet potato	
Rice biscuit	Corn pone	Lima beans	Tapioca cooked with milk and milk sugar also may be taken
Rice bread	Corn-rye muffin	Potato bread	
	Rye bread	Soybean or lima bean bread	
	Ry-Krisp		
Lettuce	Tomato	Beets	
Spinach	Squash	Carrots	
Carrot	Asparagus	Lima beans	
Beet	Peas	String beans	
Artichoke	String beans	Tomato	
Lamb	Chicken	Beef	
	Bacon	Bacon	
Lemon	Pineapple	Lemon	
Grapefruit	Peaches	Grapefruit	
Pear	Apricots	Peaches	
	Prunes	Apricots	
Cane sugar	Cane sugar	Cane sugar	
Wesson oil†	Mazola oil	Olive oil	
Olive oil	Wesson oil†	Wesson oil†	
Salt	Salt	Gelatin	
Gelatin	Karo corn syrup	Salt	
Syrup made of maple sugar or cane sugar flavored with maple‡	Gelatin	Olives	
Olives		Syrup made of maple sugar or cane sugar flavored with maple‡	
Pear butter			

*From Rowe, A. H.: Elimination diets and the patient's allergies, ed. 2, Philadelphia, 1944, Lea & Febiger.
†If patient has shown by skin test to be allergic to cottonseed, omit Wesson oil.
‡If allergy to cane sugar is suspected, use beet sugar or corn glucose.

ticular item is strongly suspected, by omitting that one item and its products from the diet.

If wheat is the suspected allergen, anything made from wheat or wheat products is omitted for at least 10 days. This means that all mixed foods must be analyzed to be certain that no wheat product is used in any preparation.

The quantity of a food that will produce allergenic symptoms varies. Also the physical condition of the patient makes a difference in the appearance of the allergy. If the individual is under strain or is overtired, he is much more likely to develop an allergic reaction to a specific food, whereas if he is rested and relaxed, he is able to tolerate it without any reaction.

Sometimes whether a food is raw or cooked makes a difference. Sometimes a person is allergic to a certain portion of the food item—for example, the white of an egg—but can tolerate the remainder. At times the mere smell of a food to which the person is allergic will cause an allergic response.

The elimination diets devised by Rowe are given in Table 24-1. Diets 1 and 2 may be used separately or together. If the patient is suspected of being sensitive to cereals, then Diet 3 should be used as the beginning diet. The beginning diet should be used at least 10 days, possibly 3 or 4 weeks, since the reacting bodies sometimes disappear very slowly. The diets must followed very carefully, and particular attention must be used in preparation of the food. Nutritive inadequacies should be guarded against. Unless the prescribed fruits and vegetables are eaten in sufficient amounts, supplementary vitamins should be taken.

When milk is excluded, meat should be eaten twice daily in order to secure adequate protein. In the absence of milk, calcium should be given in supplementary form.

It is important not to go hungry on an elimination diet. Eating solid food for breakfast is also important. One should not lose weight on the diet. Adequate portions of the foods allowed should be eaten.

Following is a list of foods permitted on a diet free of wheat, corn, milk, eggs, chicken, rye products, strong seasonings, and canned fruits except dietetic fruits labeled "without sugar."

Salt	Beef
White cane, granulated or lump, sugar	Veal
Water, freshly squeezed fruit juice, coffee made of freshly ground coffee bean, and fresh lemonade made with cane sugar	Lamb
	Turkey
	Pork chops and pork roast
All fruits (thoroughly washed)	Ham, baked, boiled, and fried
All vegetables, except corn (thoroughly washed)	Bacon and canadian bacon
	Ripe olives
White uncoated rice	Olive oil (pure)
	Walnuts and almonds in the shell

Do not eat or drink or prepare food with any ingredient that is not included in the allergy diet list. No chewing gum, candy, shortening, seasoning, frozen juices, and so forth, are permitted.

Baking soda should be used instead of tooth powder or toothpaste. One-half teaspoon of baking soda to one-half glass of lukewarm water should be used instead of mouthwash.

Breakfast could include rice, water, salt, cane sugar, banana, bacon, ham, and coffee. When eating out, one could order a vegetable plate, rice, roast beef or steaks, chops, bacon, ham, and banana or other raw fruit for dessert. For infants, as a substitute for milk, one cup of hot water may be added to one-half can of strained beef and mixed with an egg beater. This could be taken from a baby bottle.

When the period of relief from the allergy symptoms has been of sufficient duration, other foods may be cautiously added. Thereafter, canned vegetables and fruits, other meats, spices, and nuts are gradually added. After 1 to 3 months, wheat, milk, and eggs may be added, one at a time, and the results should be observed carefully. The reaction may appear immediately or several days after an article has been added to the menu.

After the person has isolated his allergies and has remained on a restricted diet for some time, he can try to desensitize himself by adding minute quantities of one allergen at a time to his diet, very gradually adding a little more of the same food until he has built up a resistance to that particular food.

Recent studies of children with learning problems and hyperkinesis have indicated a possible allergic sensitivity to salicylates and food colors and flavors used in a wide variety of foods. Some of these children have shown a rapid dramatic improvement in scholastic achievement when treated with a salicylate-free diet.

Questions on allergy

1. What is an allergen?
2. In what ways do allergens enter the body?
3. What are the food that most often cause allergic symptoms?
4. How does heredity affect the appearance of allergy?
5. In what ways does an allergen usually manifest itself in children?
6. To what foods are children most likely to be allergic?
7. If a child is allergic to cow's milk, what other types of milk can usually be given?
8. If a person is allergic to raw tomatoes, would it be possible for him to eat cooked tomatoes?
9. Plan a diet based on Rowe's Elimination Diets 1 and 2.
10. Plan a diet based on Rowe's Diet 3.

Suggestions for additional study

1. Make a report on the various ways in which food allergies can affect a person.
2. Read the labels on various cereals and determine which ones can be used on a wheat-free diet and which ones can be used on a corn-free diet.

3. A patient is on an egg-free, wheat-free diet. May he have the following foods: orange, juice, broiled lamb chop, oatmeal, ryebread, mashed potatoes, apple dumpling, baked apple, noodles, buttermilk, shredded wheat, gelatin with fruit?

References

Fiengold, B. F.: Why your child is hyperactive, New York, 1975, Random House, Inc.

Rowe, A. H.: Elimination diet and the patient's allergies, ed. 2, Philadelphia, 1944, Lea & Febiger.

Speer, F.: Food allergy, Littleton, Mass., 1979, PSG Publishing Co., Inc.

Williams, S. R.: Nutrition and diet therapy, ed. 3, St. Louis, 1977, The C. V. Mosby Co.

Williams, S. R.: Essentials of nutrition and diet therapy, ed. 2, St. Louis, 1978, The C. V. Mosby Co.

APPENDIX

Table A. Food values*

	Approximate measure	Calories	Protein (gm.)	Fat (gm.)	Carbohydrate (gm.)
Beverages					
Coca-Cola	1 bottle (6 oz.)	78	0	0	20.4
Ginger ale	1 glass (6 oz.)	60	0	0	15.3
Chocolate milk shake	1 regular (8 oz. milk)	421	11.2	17.8	58.0
Chocolate malted milk shake	1 regular (8 oz. milk)	502	13.1	19.5	72.1
Cider, sweet	1 glass (6 oz.)	94	0.2	0	25.8
Cocoa, all milk	1 cup (6 oz. milk)	174	6.9	8.5	20.3
Eggnog	1 glass (6 oz. milk)	233	12.5	12.6	17.7
Lemonade	1 large glass, 1 oz. lemon juice	104	0.2	0	27.2
Milk, buttermilk	½ pt.	86	8.5	0.2	12.4
Milk, chocolate	½ pt.	185	8.0	5.5	26.5
Milk, skim	½ pt.	87	8.6	0.2	12.5
Milk, whole	½ pt.	166	8.5	9.5	12.0
Soda, ice cream, vanilla	1 regular	261	2.3	7.1	48.7
Soda, ice cream, chocolate	1 regular	255	2.7	8.3	46.0
Breads					
Bread, corn	1 piece (2 in. square)	139	3.2	4.3	21.6
Bread, rye	1 slice	57	2.1	0.3	12.1
Bread, white, enriched	1 slice	63	2.0	0.7	11.9
Bread, whole-wheat	1 slice	55	2.1	0.6	11.3
Biscuit, baking powder	1 average (2 in. diam.)	109	2.4	4.1	14.9
Bun, cinnamon, plain	1 average	158	3.1	4.8	25.6
Doughnut, cake type, plain	1 average	135	2.2	6.5	17.5
Doughnut, sugared or iced	1 average	151	2.2	6.5	21.7
Muffin, white flour	1 average, 12 from 2 cups flour	120	3.2	4.3	17.1
Muffin, whole-wheat	1 average, 12 from 2 cups flour	120	3.4	4.3	17.1
Pancake, various flours	1 average (4 in. diam.)	62	2.3	1.2	10.7
Roll, white, soft	1 Parker House	81	2.1	1.6	13.6

*From Church, C. F., and Church, H. N.: Food values of portions commonly used, ed. 11, Phila
Abbreviations: diam., diameter; gm., gram; I.U., international unit; lb., pound; μg, microgram; mg.
data inadequate to give a specific figure; 0, none; tr., trace.
Equivalents: 1,000 micrograms (μg) = 1 milligram (mg.); 1,000 milligrams (mg.) = 1 gram (gm.);

Calcium (mg.)	Iron (mg.)	Vitamin A (I.U.)	Thiamine (μg)	Riboflavin (μg)	Niacin (mg.)	Ascorbic acid (mg.)
0	0	0	0	0	0	0
0	0	0	0	0	0	0
363	0.9	687	120	547	0.5	4
420	1.3	891	186	655	0.5	4
11	0.9	75	37	56	tr.	2
224	0.9	295	80	334	0.3	2
242	1.5	843	123	451	0.2	2
4	tr.	0	20	tr.	tr.	15
288	0.2	10	90	430	0.3	3
272	0.2	230	80	400	0.2	2
303	0.2	10	90	440	0.3	3
288	0.2	390	90	420	0.3	3
69	0.1	205	24	106	0.1	1
75	0.7	297	30	127	0.2	1
29	0.7	229	90	102	0.7	(0)
17	0.4	0	40	20	0.4	(0)
18	0.4	0	60	40	0.5	0
22	0.5	0	70	30	0.7	0
19	0.5	20	86	70	0.6	0
27	0.9	205	85	87	0.8	0
12	0.6	41	72	63	0.5	tr.
12	0.6	41	72	63	0.5	tr.
30	0.7	193	78	95	0.6	0
33	0.7	193	88	85	0.5	0
96	0.3	44	30	53	0.2	0
19	0.5	73	72	64	0.5	0

lelphia, 1970, J. B. Lippincott Co.

nilligram; oz., ounce; tbs., tablespoonful, level; tsp., teaspoonful, level; ( ), tentative data; —,

.8.34 grams = 1 oz.   *Continued.*

Table A. Food values—cont'd

	Approximate measure	Calories	Protein (gm.)	Fat (gm.)	Carbo-hydrate (gm.)
Breads—cont'd					
Roll, white, sweet	1 average commercial	178	4.7	4.3	29.6
Waffle, plain, average	1 waffle (5½ in. diam.)	232	5.1	14.0	21.4
Cereals and cereal products					
Cheerios	1 oz. (1⅛ cups)	104	4.1	2.0	19.7
Cornflakes	1 oz. (1⅓ cups)	105	2.1	0.1	24.4
Cream of Wheat, cooked	¾ cup	102	3.5	0.3	21.7
Grapenuts	1 oz. (¼ cup)	110	2.8	0.2	24.0
Macaroni, cooked	½ cup (1 in. pieces)	105	3.6	0.4	21.2
Macaroni and cheese, baked	1 cup	366	15.3	19.9	31.4
Noodles, egg, en-riched, cooked	¾ cup	81	2.7	0.75	15.3
Oatmeal, cooked	¾ cup	111	4.0	2.1	19.5
Popcorn	1 cup	54	1.8	0.7	10.7
Post Toasties	1¼ cups (1 oz.)	100	2.1	0.1	24.0
Rice, white, cooked	¾ cup	150	3.2	0.15	33.0
Rice Krispies	1 cup	107	1.6	0.1	25.1
Rice, puffed	1 cup	107	1.8	0.1	24.7
Spaghetti, cooked	¾ cup	162	5.5	0.6	33.0
Spaghetti, Italian style	1 average serving with meat sauce	396	12.7	20.7	39.4
Sugar Crisp	1 oz. (individual package)	110	1.9	0.3	25.0
Wheat, shredded	1 large biscuit (4 in. × 2¼ in.)	106	3.2	0.5	22.1
Cracker, graham	1 (2½ in. sq.)	28	0.5	0.7	5.0
Cracker, Ritz	1 cracker	16	0.2	0.8	2.0
Cracker, saltine	1 cracker	14	0.3	0.3	2.3
Matzoth	1 piece (6 in. diam.)	78	2.1	0.2	17.3
Pretzel sticks	7 average thin sticks	37	0.9	0.3	7.5
Ry-Krisp	1 double square wafer	20	0.7	0.1	4.1
Zwieback	1 piece (61 to 1 lb.)	31	0.9	0.7	5.3
Dairy products					
Butter	1 tsp.	36	0	4.1	0
Butter	1 tbs.	100	0.1	11.3	0.1
Cheese, cheddar, American	1 oz. (1 slice ¼ in. thick)	113	7.1	9.1	0.6
Cheese, cottage	½ cup	107	22.0	0.55	2.2

*Vitamin A and D values for butter and cream are average year-round figures; vitamin A and D

Calcium (mg.)	Iron (mg.)	Vitamin A (I.U.)	Thiamine (μg)	Riboflavin (μg)	Niacin (mg.)	Ascorbic acid (mg.)
35	0.3	0	30	70	0.6	0
59	0.9	178	122	159	0.8	tr.
47	2.1	(0)	325	56	0.6	0
2	0.5	(0)	120	20	0.6	0
10	1.1	0	17	17	0.2	0
—	1.0	(0)	130	—	1.5	0
7	0.75	(0)	120	75	1.0	0
355	1.2	818	96	355	0.9	tr.
4	0.6	45	165	75	1.35	0
15	1.2	(0)	165	38	0.3	0
(2)	(0.4)	(0)	(50)	(20)	(0.3)	0
—	0.4	(0)	110	—	0.5	0
9	0.4	(0)	15	7	0.5	0
7	0.5	(0)	110	10	2.0	0
4	0.5	(0)	125	11	1.5	0
10	1.2	(0)	186	113	0.5	0
27	2.1	901	120	117	3.0	(24)
3	0.5	(0)	14	—	0.7	0
13	1.0	(0)	60	30	1.3	0
1	0.1	(0)	20	10	0.1	0
1	0.1	(0)	—	—	—	0
1	0.1	(0)	tr.	tr.	tr.	0
—	—	0	—	—	—	0
1	0.1	0	1	4	0.1	0
3	0.2	0	20	10	0.1	0
8	0.1	0	—	—	—	0
1	0	165°	tr.	tr.	tr.	0
3	—	460°	tr.	tr.	tr.	0
206	0.3	400	10	120	tr.	(0)
108	0.35	25	20	345	0.1	(0)

content varies with the seasons.

Continued.

Table A. Food values—cont'd

	Approximate measure	Calories	Protein (gm.)	Fat (gm.)	Carbohydrate (gm.)
Dairy products —cont'd					
Cheese, cream	2 tbs.	106	2.6	10.5	0.6
Cream, light	1 tbs.	30	0.4	3.0	0.6
Cream, heavy, sweet or sour	1 tbs.	50	0.3	5.2	0.5
Cream, heavy, whipped	1 heaping tbs., sweetened	52	0.3	5.2	1.3
Milk, whole	½ pt.	166	8.5	9.5	12.0
Milk, chocolate	½ pt.	185	8.0	5.5	26.5
Milk, skim	½ pt.	87	8.6	0.2	12.5
Milk, buttermilk	½ pt.	86	8.5	0.2	12.4
Desserts					
Vanilla blancmange	½ cup	152	4.2	4.7	23.8
Brownies	1 (2 in. × 2 in. × ¾ in.)	141	1.8	8.4	16.6
Cake, angel	1 piece (¹/₁₀ of average cake)	145	3.4	0.1	33.0
Cake, chocolate, 2 layer	1 piece (¹/₁₂ of cake with white icing)	356	3.1	7.7	45.0
Cake, white 2 layer, chocolate icing	3 in. section of layer cake	314	4.0	10.4	52.6
Cake, sponge cake	1 piece (¹/₁₀ of average cake)	145	3.2	2.3	28.1
Cookies, oatmeal	1 large (3½ in. diam.)	114	1.6	4.4	17.5
Cookies, sugar	1 cookie (3½ in. diam.)	64	1.0	2.6	9.1
Custard, baked	1 custard (4 from 1 pt. milk)	205	8.8	9.1	22.8
Fig bars, commercial	1 small, average	56	0.7	0.8	12.1
Gingerbread, using hot water and 1 egg	1 small piece (2 in. cube)	206	2.2	9.9	26.9
Ice cream, vanilla	¼ of 1 pt.	147	2.8	8.9	14.6
Jell-O, plain	1 serving (5 to 1 package)	65	1.6	0	15.1
Jell-O with whipped cream	1 serving, 1 tbs. cream	117	1.8	5.4	16.4
Pie, apple	¹/₆ of medium pie	377	3.8	14.3	60.2
Pie, blueberry	¹/₆ of medium pie	372	3.9	15.4	56.9
Pie, cherry	¹/₆ of medium pie	360	4.3	12.4	59.6
Pie, chocolate	¹/₆ of medium pie	294	6.9	13.7	37.7
Pie, custard	¹/₆ of medium pie	266	7.6	12.1	32.7

°Vitamin A and D values for butter and cream are average year-round figures; vitamin A and D

Calcium (mg.)	Iron (mg.)	Vitamin A (I.U.)	Thiamine (μg)	Riboflavin (μg)	Niacin (mg.)	Ascorbic acid (mg.)
19	0.1	(410)	tr.	60	tr.	(0)
15	0	120°	4	20	tr.	tr.
12	0	220°	tr.	20	tr.	tr.
12	0	220°	tr.	20	tr.	tr.
288	0.2	(390)	90	420	0.3	3
272	0.2	230	80	400	0.2	2
303	0.2	(10)	90	440	0.3	3
(288)	0.2	10	90	430	0.3	1
144	0.1	195	45	210	0.1	1
11	0.5	226	38	41	0.2	(0)
3	0.1	(0)	3	66	0.1	0
24	0.5	265	17	70	0.1	(0)
88	0.4	390	20	70	0.2	(0)
12	0.6	220	24	59	0.1	(0)
12	0.5	27	59	36	0.2	(0)
5	0.2	25	32	27	0.2	(0)
163	1.1	607	82	315	0.1	(0)
11	0.2	0	3	10	0.1	(0)
45	1.4	69	66	54	0.5	0
87	0.1	369	29	135	0.1	1
(0)	(0)	(0)	(0)	(0)	(0)	(0)
12	(0)	212	4	16	tr.	tr.
11	0.5	156	46	26	0.4	1
14	0.7	166	25	29	0.4	5
16	0.6	601	41	26	0.4	2
118	0.8	325	30	128	0.2	(0)
111	0.8	305	63	215	0.2	(0)

ontent varies with the seasons.

Continued.

Table A. Food values—cont'd

		Calories	Protein (gm.)	Fat (gm.)	Carbo-hydrate (gm.)
Desserts—cont'd					
Pie, lemon meringue	¹/₆ of medium pie	281	3.8	9.8	45.3
Pie, mince	¹/₆ of medium pie	398	3.9	10.9	71.8
Pie, raisin	¹/₆ of medium pie	437	4.6	12.4	81.2
Pie, pumpkin	¹/₆ of medium pie	330	6.7	10.7	53.5
Sherbet, average	¹/₂ cup commercial	118	1.4	0	28.8
Shortcake, biscuit, strawberries	1 cup berries, 1 medium biscuit	399	4.8	8.9	61.2
Pudding, cornstarch, chocolate	¹/₂ cup	219	4.5	6.6	37.1
Pudding, cornstarch, vanilla	¹/₂ cup	152	4.2	4.7	23.8
Pudding, tapioca, cream	¹/₂ cup	133	4.9	5.0	17.3
Eggs					
Egg, cooked, boiled	1 medium	77	6.1	5.5	0.3
Egg, fried	1 medium, 1 tsp. margarine	110	6.1	9.2	0.3
Egg, omelet, plain	1 medium	120	6.6	9.8	1.0
Egg, omelet, Spanish	2 eggs, 4 tbs. sauce	329	14.6	26.9	7.6
Egg, scrambled	1 medium, 1 tbs. milk, 1 tsp. fat	120	6.6	9.8	1.0
Fats and oils					
Butter	1 tsp.	36	tr.	4.1	tr.
Butter	1 tbs.	100	0.1	11.3	0.1
Dressing, commercial mayonnaise	1 tbs.	58	0.2	5.5	2.1
Dressing, commercial French	1 tbs.	59	0.1	5.3	3.0
Dressing, homemade mayonnaise	1 tbs.	92	0.2	10.1	0.4
Dressing, homemade French	1 tbs.	86	0.0	9.2	0.7
Dressing, Thousand Island	1 rounded tbs.	98	0.3	10.0	2.4
Margarine	1 tsp.	36	tr.	4.1	tr.
Margarine	1 tbs.	100	0.1	11.3	0.1
Fish					
Flounder or sole, baked	¹/₄ lb.	204	16.9	20.0	0
Haddock, cooked, fried	1 fillet (3 in. × 3 in. × ¹/₂ in.)	214	23.5	9.0	8.1
Halibut steak, cooked	1 serving (4 to 1 lb.)	205	21.0	12.2	0
Herring, pickled	2 small	223	20.4	15.1	0
Oysters, fried	6 oysters	412	15.1	29.6	18.2

Calcium (mg.)	Iron (mg.)	Vitamin A (I.U.)	Thiamine (μg)	Riboflavin (μg)	Niacin (mg.)	Ascorbic acid (mg.)
13	0.5	260	29	52	0.1	1
35	3.4	12	106	55	0.5	1
47	2.0	27	98	53	0.5	(0)
103	2.2	2,278	58	163	0.5	(0)
48	0	0	20	70	0	(0)
73	2.0	429	167	207	1.3	(89)
147	0.2	196	45	217	0.2	(0)
144	0.1	195	45	210	0.1	(0)
105	0.5	313	46	186	0.1	1
26	1.3	550	40	130	tr.	0
27	1.3	702	40	130	tr.	0
44	1.3	726	46	153	tr.	0
103	3.4	2,008	110	260	1.0	13
44	1.3	726	56	165	tr.	0
1	0	165	tr.	tr.	tr.	0
3	0	460	tr.	tr.	tr.	0
1	0.1	20	tr.	tr.	(0)	(0)
tr.	tr.	0	0	0	0	0
2	0.1	34	3	3	tr.	0
tr.	tr.	(0)	(0)	(0)	(0)	0
3	0.2	109	9	5	0.1	1
1	0	165	(0)	(0)	(0)	(0)
3	0	460	(0)	(0)	(0)	(0)
69	0.9	–	49	54	1.6	0
44	1.4	139	69	134	2.6	–
15	0.8	497	55	61	8.8	–
22	1.1	–	–	–	–	0
134	6.4	1,539	134	274	1.2	0

Continued.

Table A. Food values—cont'd

	Approximate measure	Calories	Protein (gm.)	Fat (gm.)	Carbo-hydrate (gm.)
Fish—cont'd					
Oysters, raw	½ cup (6 to 9 medium)	100	11.8	2.5	6.7
Oysters, escalloped	1 serving 6 oysters	356	15.9	18.0	31.6
Salmon, pink	⅔ cup	143	20.5	6.2	0
Salmon, red	⅔ cup	173	20.2	9.6	0
Scallops, fried	5 to 6 medium	426	23.8	28.4	19.3
Scallops, raw	2 to 3 (12 to 1 lb.)	78	14.8	0.1	3.4
Shrimp, canned	4 to 6 shrimp	64	13.4	0.7	0
Tuna, canned	⅝ cup solids	198	29.0	8.2	0
Fruits					
Apple, baked, unpared	1 large, 2 tbs. sugar	213	0.6	0.8	64.9
Apple, raw	1 small (2¼ in. diam.)	50	0.3	0.4	13.0
Apple, raw	1 large (3 in. diam.)	117	0.6	0.8	30.1
Applesauce, canned	½ cup, sweetened	92	0.3	0.2	25.0
Applesauce, canned	½ cup	50	0.3	0.3	13.1
Apricots, raw	2 to 3 medium	51	1.0	0.1	12.9
Apricots, canned in syrup	4 halves, 2 tbs. juice	80	0.6	0.1	21.4
Apricots, canned in water	4 halves	32	0.5	0.1	8.1
Avocado	½ small pear	245	1.7	26.4	5.1
Banana, raw	1 small	88	1.2	0.2	23.0
Banana, raw	1 medium	132	1.8	0.3	34.5
Banana, raw	1 large	176	2.4	0.4	46.0
Blueberries, canned in syrup	½ cup	123	0.5	0.5	32.4
Blueberries, canned in water	½ cup	45	0.5	0.5	10.9
Blueberries, frozen, no sugar	⅝ cup	61	0.6	0.6	15.1
Cantaloupe, diced	½ cup	24	0.7	0.2	5.5
Cherries, canned, sweet, in syrup	½ cup red	105	0.6	0.1	28.5
Cherries, canned in water	½ cup red	51	0.8	0.4	12.6
Cherries, maraschino	1 cherry	19	tr.	tr.	5.2
Cranberry jelly	1 rounded tbs.	47	tr.	tr.	13.0
Cranberry sauce	1 rounded tbs.	40	tr.	0.1	10.3
Dates, dried and fresh	3 to 4 pitted	85	0.6	0.2	22.6
Figs, canned in syrup	3 figs, 2 tbs. juice	113	0.8	0.3	30.0
Figs, dried	2 small	81	1.2	0.4	20.5
Fruit cocktail, canned	6 tbs. fruit and juice	70	0.4	0.2	18.6

Calcium (mg.)	Iron (mg.)	Vitamin A (I.U.)	Thiamine (µg)	Riboflavin (µg)	Niacin (mg.)	Ascorbic acid (mg.)
113	6.7	385	175	240	1.4	–
158	7.0	894	143	277	1.5	0
187	0.8	70	30	180	8.0	(0)
259	1.2	230	40	160	7.3	(0)
41	3.1	0	91	173	2.3	(0)
26	1.8	0	(40)	100	1.4	–
58	1.6	30	5	15	1.1	(0)
(8)	1.4	80	50	120	12.8	(0)
12	0.6	(180)	40	45	0.3	(2)
5	0.3	80	33	27	0.1	4
12	0.6	180	80	60	0.4	9
5	0.5	40	25	15	0.1	1 to 2
5	0.5	35	25	10	0.1	1 to 2
16	0.5	2,790	30	50	0.8	7
10	0.3	1,350	20	20	0.3	4
10	0.3	1,350	20	20	0.3	4
10	0.6	290	60	130	1.1	16
8	0.6	430	40	50	0.7	10
12	0.9	645	60	75	1.0	15
16	1.2	860	80	100	1.4	20
14	0.6	50	15	15	0.3	17
14	0.6	50	15	15	0.3	16
16	0.8	240	20	20	0.3	14
20	0.5	4,104	60	48	0.6	40
11	0.3	430	30	20	0.1	3
11	0.3	120	30	20	0.1	3
1	tr.	35	(3)	(2)	tr.	tr.
tr.	tr.					
(2)	(0.1)	(6)	(4)	(4)	tr.	tr.
22	0.6	18	27	30	0.7	(0)
35	0.4	50	30	30	0.4	tr.
56	0.9	24	48	36	0.5	(0)
9	0.4	160	10	10	0.4	2

Continued.

Table A. Food values—cont'd

	Approximate measure	Calories	Protein (gm.)	Fat (gm.)	Carbo-hydrate (gm.)
Fruits—cont'd					
Grapefruit, raw	½ small	40	0.5	0.2	10.1
Grapefruit, raw	½ large (5 in. diam.)	100	1.3	0.5	25.3
Grapes, green seedless	60	66	0.8	0.4	16.7
Grapes, Tokay	22	66	0.8	0.4	16.7
Honeydew melon	¼ of 5 in. diam. melon	32	0.5	0	8.5
Lemons, raw	1 medium	32	0.9	0.6	8.7
Limes, raw	1 large	37	0.8	0.1	12.3
Olives, green	1 large	7	0.1	0.7	0.2
Olives, ripe	1 large or 2 small	7	0.1	0.7	0.2
Orange, whole	1 small (2½ in. diam.)	45	0.9	0.2	11.2
Orange, whole	1 large (3⅜ in diam.)	106	2.1	0.5	26.3
Orange sections	½ cup	44	0.9	0.2	10.8
Peaches, raw	1 medium large	46	0.5	0.1	12.0
Peaches, raw	1 cup, sliced	77	0.8	0.2	20.2
Peaches, canned in syrup	2 halves, 1 tbs. juice	68	0.4	0.1	18.2
Peaches, canned water-pack	2 halves, 2 tbs. juice	27	0.5	0.1	6.8
Peaches, frozen	½ cup, scant	78	0.4	0.1	20.2
Pears, raw	1 medium pear	63	0.7	0.4	15.8
Pears, canned in syrup	2 halves, 1 tbs. juice	68	0.2	0.1	18.4
Pears, canned in water	2 halves, 1 tbs. juice	31	0.3	0.1	8.2
Pineapple, canned in syrup	½ cup, crushed	102	0.5	0.2	27.5
Pineapple, canned in syrup	1 large or 2 small slices, 1 tbs. juice	78	0.4	0.1	21.1
Pineapple, canned in juice	1 large or 2 small slices, 2 tbs. juice	55	0.5	0.1	14.5
Plums, raw	2 medium	50	0.7	0.2	12.9
Plums, canned in syrup	2 medium, 2 tbs. juice	76	0.4	0.1	20.4
Prunes, dried, raw	3 medium or 4 small	67	0.6	0.2	17.8
Prunes, cooked, no sugar	4 medium, 2 tbs. juice	86	0.7	0.2	22.7
Prunes, cooked, with sugar	4 medium, 2 tbs. juice	119	0.7	0.2	31.2
Raisins, dried	1 tbs.	27	0.2	0.1	7.2
Raisins, dried	1 cup	429	3.7	0.8	113.9

Calcium (mg.)	Iron (mg.)	Vitamin A (I.U.)	Thiamine (µg)	Riboflavin (µg)	Niacin (mg.)	Ascorbic acid (mg.)
22	0.2	tr.	40	20	0.2	40
55	0.5	tr.	100	50	0.5	100
17	0.6	80	60	40	0.2	4
17	0.6	80	60	40	0.2	4
(17)	(0.4)	40	50	30	0.2	23
40	0.6	0	40	tr.	0.1	50
(40)	0.6	0	(40)	tr.	(0.1)	27
5	0.1	16	tr.	−	−	−
5	0.1	3	tr.	tr.	−	−
33	0.4	(190)	80	30	0.2	49
78	0.9	(447)	188	71	0.5	115
32	0.4	(180)	75	25	0.3	48
8	0.6	880	20	50	0.9	8
13	1.0	1,478	34	84	1.5	13
5	0.4	450	10	20	0.7	4
5	0.4	450	10	20	0.7	4
6	0.4	520	10	30	0.5	4
13	0.3	20	20	40	0.1	4
8	0.2	tr.	10	20	0.1	2
8	0.2	tr.	10	20	0.1	2
38	0.8	105	100	20	0.2	12
29	0.6	80	70	20	0.2	9
29	0.6	80	70	20	0.2	9
17	0.5	350	60	40	0.5	5
8	1.1	230	30	30	0.4	1
14	1.0	473	25	40	0.2	tr.
17	1.3	545	22	45	0.4	tr.
17	1.3	545	22	45	0.4	tr.
8	0.3	5	15	8	0.1	−
125	5.3	80	240	130	0.8	tr.

Continued.

Table A. Food values—cont'd

	Approximate measure	Calories	Protein (gm.)	Fat (gm.)	Carbo-hydrate (gm.)
Fruits—cont'd					
Raspberries, black, raw	⅔ cup	74	1.5	1.6	15.7
Raspberries, red, raw	¾ cup	57	1.2	0.4	13.8
Rhubarb, cooked, sweetened	½ cup fruit and syrup	137	0.3	0.1	35.1
Strawberries, raw	10 large	37	0.8	0.5	8.3
Strawberries, frozen, sweetened	½ cup, scant	106	0.6	0.4	26.6
Watermelon	½ cup cubes	28	0.5	0.2	6.9
Watermelon	1 slice (6 in. diam., 1½ in. thick)	168	3.0	1.2	41.4
Fruit juices					
Apple juice, canned	2 tbs.	16	0.03	0	4.3
Apple juice, canned	3 fl. oz.	48	0.1	0	13.8
Apricot juice	3 fl. oz.	44	0.5	0.4	10.2
Grape juice, commercial	3 fl. oz.	67	0.4	0	18.2
Grapefruit juice, fresh	3¼ fl. oz.	36	0.5	0.1	9.2
Grapefruit juice, canned	3¼ fl. oz. sweetened	52	0.5	0.1	13.7
Grapefruit juice, canned	3¼ fl. oz.	38	0.5	0.1	9.8
Lemon juice, fresh	1 tbs.	4	0.1	tr.	1.2
Orange juice, fresh	3¼ fl. oz.	44	0.8	0.2	11.0
Orange juice, canned	3¼ fl. oz. sweetened	54	0.6	0.2	13.9
Orange juice, canned	3⅛ fl. oz.	44	0.8	0.2	11.1
Pineapple juice, canned	3¼ fl. oz.	49	0.3	0.1	13.0
Prune juice, canned	3 fl. oz.	63	0.3	0	17.4
Tomato juice, canned	3 fl. oz.	21	0.9	0.2	4.3
Meats					
Bacon	1 strip, drained (6 in.)	48	1.8	4.4	0.2
Bacon, Canadian, cooked	1 slice (2¼ in. diam., 3⁄16 in. thick)	57	6.6	3.1	0.1
Beef brisket, raw	3 pieces (2 in. × 1 in. × 1 in.)	338	15.8	30.0	0
Beef, chuck, pot roast	1 slice (2 in. × 1½ in. × ½ in.)	93	7.8	6.6	0
Beef, hamburger, average cooked	1 small patty (2 oz.)	118	12.9	7.1	0
Beef, hamburger, average cooked	1 medium patty (5 to 1 lb.)	246	14.6	20.4	0

*Calcium may not be available because of high oxalic acid content.

Calcium (mg.)	Iron (mg.)	Vitamin A (I.U.)	Thiamine (μg)	Riboflavin (μg)	Niacin (mg.)	Ascorbic acid (mg.)
40	0.9	0	20	(70)	(0.3)	(24)
40	0.9	130	20	(70)	(0.3)	24
26°	0.2	16	2	–	tr.	2
28	0.8	60	30	70	0.3	60
22	0.6	40	20	50	0.2	41
7	0.2	590	50	50	0.2	6
42	1.2	3,540	300	300	1.2	36
2	0.2	12	6	9	tr.	tr.
6	0.5	40	20	30	tr.	1
10	0.3	–	40	50	0.2	tr.
8	0.3	tr.	40	20	0.2	40
8	0.3	tr.	30	20	0.2	35
8	0.3	tr.	30	20	0.2	35
2	tr.	0	6	tr.	tr.	8
19	0.2	(190)	80	30	0.2	40
10	0.3	(100)	70	20	0.2	42
10	0.3	(100)	70	20	0.2	42
15	0.5	80	50	20	0.2	9
(24)	(1.5)	–	27	72	0.3	tr.
(6)	(0.3)	978	48	27	0.6	15
3	0.2	(0)	40	22	0.3	0
4	1.0	(0)	164	67	1.4	0
0	2.4	(0)	100	130	4.4	0
3	0.9	(0)	15	60	1.2	0
7	1.9	(0)	38	102	2.6	0
8	2.2	0	43	115	3.0	0

Continued.

Table A. Food values—cont'd

	Approximate measure	Calories	Protein (gm.)	Fat (gm.)	Carbo-hydrate (gm.)
Meats—cont'd					
Beef, hamburger, average cooked	1 large patty (4 to 1 lb.)	300	18.2	24.6	0
Beef, hamburger on bun	1 average, plain	332	17.1	21.9	15.4
Beef, porterhouse, broiled	1 large steak with gravy (5 oz.)	513	34.5	40.5	0
Beef, rib, roasted	1 slice (3 in. × 2¼ in. × ¼ in.)	96	7.2	7.2	0
Beef, round, cubed, cooked	1 piece, 3 oz. (4 in. × 3 in. × ⅜ in.)	214	24.7	12.0	0
Beef, rump, pot roast	1 slice (5 in. × 3½ in. × ¼ in.)	320	17.8	27.2	0
Beef steak, club broiled	1 large (4 oz.)	410	27.6	32.4	0
Beef stew with potatoes, carrots, onions, gravy	3 oz. chuck, 2 small potatoes, 1 small carrot, 1 onion	529	28.1	19.6	56.1
Beef tongue, medium cooked	3 slices, 2 oz. (3 in. × 2 in. × ⅛ in.)	160	11.6	12.2	0.2
Chili con carne (no beans)	½ cup, scant, 60% meat	200	10.3	14.8	5.8
Frankfurter, cooked	1 average (5½ in. long × ¾ in. diam.)	124	7.0	10.0	1.0
Ham, smoked, cooked	1 slice, 1 oz. (4 in. × 2½ in. × ⅛ in.)	119	6.9	9.9	(0.1)
Lamb chop, rib, cooked	1 chop	128	7.9	(10.5)	0
Lamb, ground, cooked	1 patty, 2 oz. (2 in. diam., ½ in. thick)	130	8.2	10.5	0
Lamb, leg, roasted	1 slice, 1 oz. (3 in. × 2¾ in. × ⅛ in.)	82	7.2	5.7	0
Liver, beef, fried	1 slice, 1½ oz. (3 in. × 2¼ in. × ⅜ in.)	86	8.8	2.9	5.6
Liver, calf, cooked	1 slice, 1⅓ oz. (3 in. × 2¼ in. × ⅜ in.)	74	8.1	3.6	1.7
Liver, chicken, cooked	1 medium large liver	74	8.8	3.6	1.0
Meat loaf, beef and pork	1 slice, 2⅓ oz. (4 in. × 3 in. × ⅜ in.)	264	10.4	19.2	11.5
Meat gravy	1 tbs.	41	0.3	3.5	2.0
Pork chop, loin, fried	1 medium (2⅓ oz.)	233	16.1	18.2	0
Pork, loin, roasted	1 slice, 1 oz. (3 in. × 2½ in. × ¼ in.)	100	6.9	7.8	0
Pork, spareribs, roasted	Meat from 6 average ribs (3 oz.)	246	15.4	(20.0)	0
Veal chop, loin, fried	1 medium (3 oz.)	186	21.8	9.4	0

Calcium (mg.)	Iron (mg.)	Vitamin A (I.U.)	Thiamine (μg)	Riboflavin (μg)	Niacin (mg.)	Ascorbic acid (mg.)
11	2.7	0	54	144	3.7	0
23	2.4	0	63	145	3.3	0
17	4.5	(0)	90	270	7.1	0
3	0.9	(0)	18	54	1.9	0
10	3.1	(0)	74	202	5.1	0
7	2.1	(0)	34	128	2.6	0
13	3.6	(0)	72	216	5.6	0
86	5.0	5,590	255	280	5.5	(20)
4	(1.5)	(0)	(30)	(130)	(1.5)	0
38	1.4	150	20	120	2.2	0
3	0.6	(0)	80	90	1.2	0
3	0.9	(0)	162	63	1.3	0
4	1.1	(0)	45	80	1.9	0
4	1.0	(0)	85	150	2.7	0
3	0.9	(0)	42	75	1.5	0
4	2.9	18,658	90	1,283	5.1	(10)
3	4.5	9,565	63	1,193	5.9	(8)
6	3.0	12,880	56	886	4.7	(4)
26	1.7	50	118	111	2.0	(0)
tr.	(0.1)	0	(10)	(7)	tr.	—
8	2.1	(0)	580	168	3.5	(0)
3	0.9	(0)	249	72	1.5	0
8	2.2	(0)	400	150	2.8	0
10	3.0	(0)	110	265	6.7	0

Continued.

Table A. Food values—cont'd

	Approximate measure	Calories	Protein (gm.)	Fat (gm.)	Carbo-hydrate (gm.)
Meats—cont'd					
Veal cutlet, breaded, baked	1 average serving, 3 oz.	217	23.8	9.4	8.0
Veal, leg, roasted	1 slice, 1 oz. (3 in. × 2 in. × $\frac{1}{8}$ in.)	70	8.4	3.8	0
Veal, stew, carrots, onions	$\frac{1}{2}$ cup	121	8.8	7.8	3.6
Sausages					
Bologna	1 slice, 1 oz. ($4\frac{1}{2}$ in. diam., $\frac{1}{8}$ in. thick)	66	4.4	4.8	1.1
Liver sausage	1 slice, 1 oz. (3 in. diam., $\frac{1}{4}$ in. thick)	79	5.0	6.2	0.5
Luncheon meat	1 slice (1 oz.)	81	4.6	6.8	0.5
Salami	1 slice, 1 oz. ($3\frac{3}{4}$ in. diam., $\frac{1}{4}$ in. thick)	130	7.2	11.0	0
Nuts					
Almonds, chocolate	5 medium	84	2.0	6.9	5.1
Cashew nuts, roasted	6 to 8 nuts	88	2.8	7.2	4.1
Coconut, shredded, dried	2 tbs.	83	0.5	5.9	8.0
Peanut butter	1 tbs., scant	86	4.0	7.2	3.2
Peanuts, roasted	15 to 17 nuts	84	4.0	6.6	3.5
Pecans, shelled	12 halves or 2 tbs., chopped	104	1.4	11.0	2.0
Poultry					
Chicken, broiler, fried	$\frac{1}{4}$ chicken, no bone	232	22.4	13.6	3.1
Chicken, canned	$\frac{1}{3}$ cup boned meat	169	25.	6.8	0
Chicken, creamed	$\frac{1}{2}$ cup, scant	208	17.6	12.1	6.6
Chicken, fryer, fried	$\frac{1}{2}$ breast (4 oz. raw)	232	26.8	11.9	3.1
Chicken, fryer, leg, fried	1 small leg	64	10.5	5.3	1.5
Chicken, hen, stewed	1 medium thigh or $\frac{1}{2}$ breast	207	26.5	10.4	0
Chicken pie with peas, potatoes	2 in. square serving 4 oz.)	230	9.6	12.1	20.2
Chicken, roasted	3 slices ($3\frac{1}{2}$ in. × $2\frac{1}{2}$ in. × $\frac{1}{4}$ in.)	198	28.3	(8.6)	0
Duck, roasted	3 slices ($3\frac{1}{2}$ in. × 3 in. × $\frac{1}{4}$ in.)	310	22.8	23.6	0
Goose	3 slices ($3\frac{1}{2}$ in. × 3 in. × $\frac{1}{4}$ in.)	322	28.1	22.4	0
Turkey	3 slices ($3\frac{1}{2}$ in. × $2\frac{1}{2}$ in. × $\frac{1}{4}$ in.)	200	30.9	(7.6)	0

Calcium (mg.)	Iron (mg.)	Vitamin A (I.U.)	Thiamine (μg)	Riboflavin (μg)	Niacin (mg.)	Ascorbic acid (mg.)
22	3.0	(0)	102	256	6.5	0
4	1.1	(0)	40	95	2.4	0
16	1.5	1,627	34	83	1.5	(0)
(3)	1.6	(0)	54	57	0.8	0
3	1.6	1,725	51	36	1.4	(0)
6	0.4	(0)	110	54	1.1	(0)
4	1.1	(0)	75	63	0.9	0
28	0.5	0	(27)	(75)	(0.5)	tr.
7	0.8	—	95	29	0.3	0
6	0.5	0	tr.	tr.	tr.	(0)
11	0.3	0	18	20	2.4	(0)
11	0.3	0	45	20	2.4	(0)
11	0.4	8	108	17	0.1	tr.
18	1.8	230	74	168	9.7	(0)
12	1.5	(0)	32	136	5.4	0
83	1.1	328	(40)	180	3.8	tr.
19	1.3	460	67	101	10.2	0
9	1.0	161	43	113	2.4	0
16	1.6	(0)	52	150	6.0	(0)
19	1.2	143	87	68	2.3	(6)
20	2.1	(0)	80	180	9.0	(0)
19	5.8	(0)				
10	4.6	(0)				
30	5.1	0 to 20	81	173	9.8	0

Continued.

Table A. Food values—cont'd

	Approximate measure	Calories	Protein (gm.)	Fat (gm.)	Carbo-hydrate (gm.)
Salads					
Cabbage slaw	⅔ cup	68	2.3	3.5	7.9
Carrot and raisin	3 heaping tbs., lettuce leaf	153	1.9	5.8	27.9
Chicken with celery	½ cup, lettuce leaf	185	16.1	10.9	5.7
Gelatin with fruit	1 square, ¼ head lettuce	139	2.1	5.7	21.6
Gelatin with chopped vegetables	1 square, ¼ head lettuce	115	2.2	5.7	15.1
Lettuce with French dressing	1 wedge	133	1.4	10.8	6.9
Potato with onion, parsley	½ cup potato with French dressing	184	1.9	10.8	21.2
Prunes, stuffed with peanut butter	4 prunes	414	13.4	28.5	32.9
Sandwiches					
Bacon, lettuce, and tomato	1 sandwich	282	6.3	15.6	28.8
Cream cheese and jelly	1 sandwich	368	6.6	16.0	50.4
Chicken, hot with gravy	1 sandwich, 3 tbs. gravy	356	21.9	15.3	29.8
Chicken salad	1 sandwich	245	14.3	8.6	26.6
Chicken, sliced, lettuce	1 sandwich	303	15.8	14.4	26.6
Club (bacon, chicken, and tomato)	1 average, 3 slices toast, lettuce	590	35.6	20.8	41.7
Egg salad on white bread	1 average	279	10.5	12.5	30.6
Peanut butter	1 average	328	11.8	19.5	30.0
Roast beef, hot with gravy	1 average, 3 tbs. gravy	429	19.3	24.5	29.8
Tuna fish salad	1 average, white bread	278	11.0	14.2	25.8
Soups					
Asparagus, cream (Campbell's)	⅞ cup (3 to 1 can)	131	5.9	6.4	12.8
Bean, homemade	¾ cup	195	6.1	11	18.6
Beef, noodle (Campbell's)	⅞ cup	52	3.3	2.4	4.5
Celery, cream (Campbell's)	⅞ cup	146	4.9	8.6	12.2
Chicken, cream (Campbell's)	⅞ cup	145	6.5	9.9	7.7
Chicken, gumbo (Campbell's)	⅞ cup	51	1.9	0.9	8.8

Calcium (mg.)	Iron (mg.)	Vitamin A (I.U.)	Thiamine (μg)	Riboflavin (μg)	Niacin (mg.)	Ascorbic acid (mg.)
53	0.5	200	50	85	0.2	(12)
48	1.5	4,708	83	81	0.5	(6)
32	1.3	290	53	130	3.4	(5)
23	0.5	391	42	50	0.3	16
24	0.5	1,977	37	58	0.3	(8)
22	0.5	540	40	80	0.2	8
21	0.8	243	70	38	0.8	(16)
63	2.3	800	110	140	7.9	5
53	1.5	870	160	142	1.6	13
60	1.1	575	120	140	1.0	2
49	2.4	(0)	178	209	6.5	0
50	1.5	10	142	140	3.2	1
52	1.8	320	162	172	4.6	2
103	4.3	1,705	384	410	10.2	27
68	2.4	580	160	210	1.0	2
61	1.0	165	96	80	5.4	(0)
43	2.9	(0)	166	209	4.9	(0)
48	1.2	231	142	113	4.1	1
(126)	(0.1)	(171)	(40)	(182)	(0.1)	(1)
52	1.9	1,364	120	70	0.5	(0)
(126)	(0.1)	(171)	(40)	(182)	(0.1)	(1)
(126)	(0.1)	(171)	(43)	(182)	(0.1)	(1)

Continued.

Table A. Food values—cont'd

	Approximate measure	Calories	Protein (gm.)	Fat (gm.)	Carbo-hydrate (gm.)
Soups—cont'd					
Chicken, noodle (Campbell's)	⅞ cup	56	3.1	19.0	6.6
Chicken, rice (Campbell's)	⅞ cup	36	2.7	1.3	3.5
Clam chowder (Campbell's)	⅞ cup	64	2.2	2.4	8.3
Green pea (Campbell's)	⅞ cup	110	5.4	1.9	17.9
Oyster stew, home-made	1 serving, 8 oz. milk, 4 oysters	321	15.0	22.2	15.7
Scotch broth (Campbell's)	⅞ cup	96	5.8	2.8	11.8
Split pea, homemade	1 serving, ¾ cup	201	7.1	11.1	19.4
Tomato (Campbell's)	⅞ cup	141	5.6	6.1	15.9
Vegetable (Campbell's)	⅞ cup	68	2.9	1.5	10.9
Vegetable, beef (Campbell's)	⅞ cup	77	5.9	2.1	7.9
Syrups and sugars					
Honey, strained	1 tbs.	62	0.1	0	16.7
Molasses	1 tbs.	50	—	0	13.0
Sorghum syrup	1 tbs.	52	—	0	13.4
Sugar, brown	1 tbs.	52	(0)	0	13.4
Sugar, powdered	1 tbs.	42	(0)	0	10.9
Sugar, white, granulated	1 tbs.	48	(0)	0	12.4
Sweets					
Caramels, plain	1 medium	42	0.3	1.2	7.8
Chocolate creams	1 average (35 to 1 lb.)	51	0.5	1.8	9.4
Chocolate fudge, milk	1 piece 1¼ in. square (15 to 1 lb.)	118	0.5	3.1	23.7
Chocolate mints	1 medium (20 to 1 lb.)	87	0.9	3.1	15.8
Gumdrops	1 large or 8 small	33	0	0	8.6
Hershey's milk chocolate	1 bar, plain, small (1 oz.)	154	2.4	9.5	15.8
Hershey's Mr. Goodbar	1 bar	158	4.2	10.4	12.9
Jelly beans	10 jelly beans	66	0	0	16.7
Mars, Candy Bar	1 bar, 1⅜ oz.	177	2.4	8.3	24.2
Mars, Forever Yours	1 bar	122	1.1	1.6	26.7
Mars, Milky Way	1 bar	121	1.2	2.0	24.8
Mars, Snickers	1 bar	122	1.9	3.0	22.8

Calcium (mg.)	Iron (mg.)	Vitamin A (I.U.)	Thiamine (μg)	Riboflavin (μg)	Niacin (mg.)	Ascorbic acid (mg.)
352	3.8	1,058	188	550	1.1	(3)
44	1.6	1,446	139	81	1.0	(2)
(126)	(0.1)	(171)	(43)	(182)	(0.1)	(1)
1	0.2	(0)	tr.	10	tr.	1
33	0.9	—	14	12	tr.	—
30	2.4	—	—	—	—	—
11	0.4	(0)	(0)	(0)	(0)	(0)
—	—	(0)	(0)	(0)	(0)	(0)
—	—	(0)	(0)	(0)	(0)	(0)
13	0.2	17	2	14	tr.	tr.
—	—	—	—	—	—	—
14	0.2	64	3	19	tr.	tr.
—	—	—	—	—	—	—
(0)	(0)	0	0	0	0	0
57	0.7	43	27	145	0.1	tr.
34	0.5	36	47	72	2.0	tr.
52	0.4	0	17	121	0.27	tr.
22	0.2	0	15	53	0.14	tr.
29	0.2	0	15	107	0.13	tr.
27	0.1	0	10	102	0.08	tr.

Continued.

Table A. Food values—cont'd

	Approximate measure	Calories	Protein (gm.)	Fat (gm.)	Carbo-hydrate (gm.)
Sweets — cont'd					
Mars, Three Musketeers	1 bar	147	0.8	0.9	35.1
Marshmallow, plain	1 average (60 to 1 lb.)	25	0.2	0	6.2
Mints, cream	10 mints (½ in. cubes)	53	0	0	13.7
Peanut brittle	1 piece (2½ in. × 2½ in. × ⅜ in.)	110	2.1	3.9	18.2
Preserves and Jellies					
Assorted jams, commercial	1 tbs.	55	0.1	0.1	14.2
Assorted jellies	1 tbs.	50	0	0	13.0
Vegetables					
Asparagus, canned, green	6 medium stalks	21	2.4	0.2	3.9
Beans, dry with pork and tomato sauce	½ cup	147	7.5	2.7	24.0
Beans, green limas, cooked	½ cup	76	4.0	0.3	14.7
Beans, green limas, frozen	½ cup	109	6.4	0.7	19.9
Beans, green, canned	1 cup	27	1.8	0.2	5.9
Beans, green, frozen	½ cup	35	2.4	0.2	7.7
Beans, yellow, canned	1 cup	27	1.8	0.2	5.9
Beets, canned	½ cup	34	0.8	0.1	8.1
Broccoli, cooked	⅔ cup	29	3.3	0.2	5.5
Brussels sprouts, cooked	½ cup (5 to 6)	33	3.1	0.4	6.2
Cabbage, raw	½ cup	12	0.7	0.1	2.7
Cabbage, cooked	½ cup	20	1.2	0.2	4.5
Carrots, cooked	½ cup	35	0.6	0.5	7.5
Cauliflower, cooked	½ cup	15	1.5	0.1	3.0
Celery, raw	1 large outer stalk (8 in. long)	7	0.5	0.1	1.5
Celery, raw	1 cup, diced	18	1.3	0.2	3.7
Celery, cooked	½ cup	12	0.9	0.2	2.4
Corn, canned	½ cup	70	2.3	0.6	16.7
Cucumber, raw	½ medium (6 to 8 slices)	6	0.4	0	1.4
Garlic bulbs, peeled	5 bulbs	9	0.4	tr.	2.0
Kale, cooked	½ cup	20	2.0	0.3	3.6
Lettuce wedge	Small	15	1.0	0.3	2.7
Mushroom, fresh	10 small or 4 large	16	2.4	0.3	4.0
Mushroom, canned	½ cup	14	1.7	0.3	4.5
Parsley, raw	10 small sprigs	5	0.4	0.1	0.9

°Calcium may not be available due to presence of oxalic acid.

Calcium (mg.)	Iron (mg.)	Vitamin A (I.U.)	Thiamine (μg)	Riboflavin (μg)	Niacin (mg.)	Ascorbic acid (mg.)
15	0.2	0	6	43	0.04	tr.
(0)	(0)	(0)	(0)	(0)	0	0
10	0.5	7	22	12	1.2	0
2	0.1	2	4	4	0.04	1
(2)	(0.1)	(2)	(4)	(4)	(0.04)	1
23	2.1	760	90	120	1.1	18
53	2.3	110	165	45	0.6	3
23	1.4	230	110	70	0.9	12
53	1.9	220	100	70	0.8	17
45	2.1	620	40	70	0.5	7
65	1.1	450	70	100	0.6	11
45	2.1	150	40	70	0.5	7
18	0.6	15	15	35	0.2	5
130	1.3	3,400	70	150	0.8	74
24	0.9	280	28	84	0.4	33
23	0.3	40	30	25	0.2	25
39	0.4	75	40	40	0.3	27
27	0.8	14,760	30	25	0.4	3
13	0.7	54	35	50	0.3	17
20	0.2	0	20	20	0.2	3
50	0.5	0	50	40	0.4	7
33	0.3	0	25	20	0.2	3
4	0.5	190	30	50	0.8	5
5	0.2	0	20	20	0.1	4
1	0.2	–	–	–	–	3
113	1.1	4,190	35	115	0.9	26
22	0.5	540	40	80	0.2	8
9	1.0	0	100	440	4.9	5
(9)	(1.0)	0	20	300	2.4	(0)
19°	0.4	823	11	28	0.1	19

Continued.

Table A. Food values—cont'd

	Approximate measure	Calories	Protein (gm.)	Fat (gm.)	Carbo-hydrate (gm.)
Vegetables—cont'd					
Parsnips, cooked	½ cup	47	0.8	0.4	10.7
Peas, green, cooked	½ cup	73	3.6	0.5	13.8
Peppers, green, raw	1 tbs. chopped	3	0.1	tr.	0.6
Pepper, shell, baked	1 shell, no filling	17	0.8	0.1	3.9
Pickles, sour	1 large, (4 in. diam. × 1¾ in.)	15	0.7	0.3	3.0
Pickles, sweet	1 pickle (2 in. × ⅝ in.)	11	0.1	tr.	2.6
Pimento, canned	1 medium	9	0.3	0.2	2.0
Potatoes, white, baked	1 medium (2½ in. diam.)	98	2.4	0.1	22.5
Potatoes, white, boiled	1 medium (2¼ in. diam.)	83	2.0	0.1	19.1
Potatoes, white, french fried	10 pieces (2 in. × ½ in. × ½ in.)	197	2.7	9.6	26.0
Potatoes, white, mashed with milk and margarine	½ cup	123	2.1	6.0	15.9
Potato chips	10 pieces (2 in. diam.)	108	1.3	7.4	9.8
Radish, red, raw	1 small	2	0.1	tr.	0.4
Sauerkraut, canned	⅔ cup	22	1.4	0.3	4.4
Spinach	½ cup	23	2.8	0.6	3.3
Squash, summer, cooked	½ cup, scant	16	0.6	0.1	3.9
Squash, winter, baked	½ cup	47	1.9	0.4	11.0
Sweet potatoes, baked	1 medium, peeled (5 in. × 2 in.)	183	2.6	1.1	41.3
Sweet potatoes, candied	1 half (3¾ in. × 2¼ in.)	358	3.0	7.2	72.4
Tomatoes, raw	1 small	20	1.0	0.3	4.0
Tomatoes, canned	½ cup	23	1.2	0.2	4.7
Tomato catsup	1 tbs.	17	0.3	0.1	4.2
Miscellaneous					
Cocoa, dry	1 tbs.	21	(0.6)	1.7	3.4
Cornstarch	1 tbs.	29	0	0	7.0
Gelatin, dry, plain	1 tbs.	34	8.6	0	0
Postum	1 tsp.	4	0.06	tr.	0.8
Tapioca	1 tbs.	36	0.06	tr.	8.6
Alcoholic beverages†				Alco-holic grams	
Beer, average	8 oz.	112	1.4	8.9	10.6

°Calcium may not be available due to presence of oxalic acid.

†Calories in the alcoholic beverages are derived from the alcohol content.

Calcium (mg.)	Iron (mg.)	Vitamin A (I.U.)	Thiamine (µg)	Riboflavin (µg)	Niacin (mg.)	Ascorbic acid (mg.)
44	0.6	0	45	80	0.1	10
26	1.7	535	95	50	0.8	8
1	tr.	63	4	7	tr.	12
7	0.3	481	26	46	0.3	64
34	1.6	420	tr.	90	tr.	8
2	0.1	11	(0)	2	tr.	1
2	0.5	805	7	21	0.1	33
13	0.8	20	110	50	1.4	17
11	0.7	20	90	30	1.0	14
15	1.0	25	90	55	1.7	14
37	0.6	260	80	50	0.8	7
(6)	(0.4)	(10)	(40)	(20)	(0.6)	2
4	0.1	3	3	2	tr.	8
36	(0.5)	40	30	60	0.1	16
111°	1.8	10,600	70	180	0.6	27
15	0.4	260	40	70	0.6	11
24	0.8	6,190	50	150	0.6	7
44	1.1	11,410	120	80	0.9	28
72	1.8	12,500	80	80	1.0	18
11	0.6	1,100	60	40	0.5	23
(13)	0.7	1,260	72	36	0.8	19
2	0.1	(320)	15	12	0.4	2
9°	0.8	2	8	27	0.2	(0)
(0)	(0)	(0)	(0)	(0)	(0)	(0)
(0)	(0)	(0)	(0)	(0)	(0)	(0)
1	tr.	—	—	—	—	—
1	0.1	(0)	(0)	(0)	(0)	(0)
10	0.0	(0)	tr.	72	0.5	0

Continued.

Table A. Food values—cont'd

	Approximate measure	Calories	Protein (gm.)	Alcoholic (gm.)	Carbohydrate (gm.)
Alcoholic beverages —cont'd					
Eggnog, Christmas type	1 punch cup	335	3.9	15.0	18.0
Gin, dry	1 jigger (1½ oz.)	105	–	15.1	
Highball	1 glass	166	–	24.0	
Manhattan	1 cocktail	164	tr.	19.2	7.9
Martini	1 cocktail	140	0.1	18.5	0.3
Old-fashioned	1 glass	179	–	24.0	3.5
Rum	1 jigger (1½ oz.)	105	–	15.1	0
Tom Collins	1 cocktail	180	–	21.5	9.0
Whiskey, bourbon	1 jigger (1½ oz.)	119	–	17.2	0
Whiskey, Scotch	1 jigger (1½ oz.)	105	–	15.1	0
Wine, California, red	1 wine glass (3⅓ oz.)	72	0.2	10.0	0.5
Wine, port	1 wine glass (3⅓ oz.)	158	0.2	15.0	14.0

Table B. Estimated safe and adequate daily dietary intakes of additional selected

	Age (yr.)	Vitamins			Trace elements[b]	
		Vitamin K (μg)	Biotin (μg)	Pantothenic acid (mg.)	Copper (mg.)	Manganese (mg.)
Infants	0-0.5	12	35	2	0.5-0.7	0.5-0.7
	0.5-1	10-20	50	3	0.7-1.0	0.7-1.0
Children	1-3	15-30	65	3	1.0-1.5	1.0-1.5
and	4-6	20-40	85	3-4	1.5-2.0	1.5-2.0
Adolescents	7-10	30-60	120	4-5	2.0-2.5	2.0-3.0
	11+	50-100	100-200	4-7	2.0-3.0	2.5-5.0
Adults		70-140	100-200	4-7	2.0-3.0	2.5-5.0

[a]Because there is less information on which to base allowances, these figures are not given in the main table
Dietary Allowances, Revised 1979. Food and Nutrition Board, National Academy of Sciences-National Re-
[b]Since the toxic levels for many trace elements may be only several times usual intakes, the upper level

Calcium (mg.)	Iron (mg.)	Vitamin A (I.U.)	Thiamine (μg)	Riboflavin (μg)	Niacin (mg.)	Ascorbic acid (mg.)
44	0.7	84	35	113	tr.	tr.
—	—	—	—	—	—	—
—	—	—	—	—	—	—
1	tr.	35	3	2	tr.	(0)
5	0.1	4	tr.	tr.	tr.	(0)
—	—	—	—	—	—	—
—	—	—	—	—	—	—
—	—	—	—	—	—	—
—	—	—	—	—	—	—
—	—	—	—	—	—	—

vitamins and minerals[a]

	Trace elements[b]				Electrolytes		
Fluoride (mg.)	Chromium (mg.)	Selenium (mg.)	Molybdenum (mg.)	Sodium (mg.)	Potassium (mg.)	Chloride (mg.)
0.1-0.5	0.01-0.04	0.01-0.04	0.03-0.06	115-350	350-925	275-700
0.2-1.0	0.02-0.06	0.02-0.06	0.04-0.08	250-750	425-1275	400-1200
0.5-1.5	0.02-0.08	0.02-0.08	0.05-0.1	325-975	550-1650	500-1500
1.0 2.5	0.03 0.12	0.03-0.12	0.06-0.15	450-1350	775-2325	700-2100
1.5-2.5	0.05-0.2	0.05-0.2	0.1-0.3	600-1800	1000-3000	925-2775
1.5-2.5	0.05-0.2	0.05-0.2	0.15-0.5	900-2700	1525-4575	1400-4200
1.5-4.0	0.05-0.2	0.05-0.2	0.15-0.5	1100-3300	1875-5625	1700-5100

of the RDA and are provided here in the form of ranges of recommended intakes. From Recommended
search Council, Washington, D.C.
for the trace elements given in this table should not be habitually exceeded.

Glossary*

Nutrition

absorption process by which food is transferred from the digestive system to the blood.

accelerate to increase the speed.

accessory something joined to or added to another product but not essentially a part of it.

acid-base balance a balance between the acid and basic elements due partly to the balance between the intake of foods that leave an acid ash and those that leave an alkaline ash in the body.

acidosis an abnormal state in which the blood and body tissues become excessively acid.

additives elements that are added to a natural food.

adolescence the period between childhood and maturity.

alkaline medium a medium that is alkaline, as opposed to an acid medium.

amenities acceptable social behavior.

atherosclerosis fat deposits in the walls of the arteries, usually in older persons.

bacteria one-cell vegetable microorganisms concerned with fermentation and putrefaction.

basal metabolism the minimal amount of energy or number of calories needed to support the basic metabolic processes of a person at rest and 12 hours after taking food.

biological value how useful a nutrient is to the body for maintenance or growth.

calorie, large the amount of heat required to raise 1 kg. of water 1°C.; the calorie of this unit value is used in all the discussions and calculations in this text.

capillary minute blood vessel carrying blood and forming a part of the capillary system.

caries decay of bone or tooth tissue.

cartilage a translucent elastic tissue commonly called a gristle.

cell a small mass of protoplasm bounded externally by a semipermeable membrane.

cellular debris waste matter resulting from the breaking down of cells.

choline a decomposition product of lecithin essential for functioning of the liver.

colon the large intestine from the cecum to the rectum.

compound a substance composed of definite proportions of two or more elements.

---

*The following were used as references: Webster's New International Dictionary of the English Language (unabridged), ed. 2, Springfield, Mass., 1950, G. & C. Merriam Co.; Taber's Cyclopedic Medical Dictionary, ed. 6, 1953; College Standard Dictionary, New York, 1942, Funk & Wagnalls.

concentrate condensed amount of certain nutrients.

condiment an ingredient added to food to enhance the flavor of the food.

conjunctivitis inflammation of the mucous membrane that lines the eyelids and covers the exposed surface of the eyeball.

contamination the process of rendering food or water unfit for use.

cortisone a hormone from the adrenal cortex.

creatine a colorless, crystalline substance that can be isolated from various animal organs and body fluids.

culture a medium prepared in the laboratory in which to grow microorganisms.

deficiency disease a disease due to the lack of essential constituents in the diet or to defective metabolism.

duodenum the first part of the small intestine.

emulsified the combination of two liquids not mutually soluble.

endocrine pertaining to a gland that produces an internal secretion.

enzyme a chemical substance that acts upon other substances and accelerates the specific chemical reation but does not itself become a part of the final product.

facilitate to make less difficult.

fetal pertaining to the product of conception during the last 6 months of pregnancy.

fortified foods foods with additions made to give increased nutritional value.

geriatrics study and treatment of the diseases of old age.

glycogen the form in which carbohydrate is stored in the animal body for future conversion into sugar, and for subsequent use in performing muscular work or for liberating heat.

grams 28.3 grams equal 1 ounce; for practical purposes in calculating diets, 30 grams are considered equal to 1 ounce.

granule a small grainlike body.

homogenize a process that breaks up the fat globules in milk.

hormone a chemical substance that originates in a specific organ or gland in the body and is conveyed through the blood to another part of the body, stimulating it to activity.

hypoglycemia deficiency of sugar in the blood.

insecticide an agent or preparation for killing insects.

lacteal an intestinal lymphatic that conveys the chyle to the lymph circulation.

lubricant an agent that produces smoothness.

malformation abnormal shape or structure.

mammary pertaining to the breast.

metabolism the changes that foods undergo after absorption from the digestive tract.

milligram (mg.) $1/1000$ of a gram.

molecule the smallest quantity into which a substance may be divided without the loss of its characteristics.

mucus a viscid fluid secreted by mucous membranes and glands.

nonconductor a substance that does not transmit heat or electricity.
nutrients foods that supply the body with necessary elements.

optimum amounts amounts producing the best results.
organic pertaining to the internal organs of the body.
oxidation process by which a substance is combined with oxygen.
oxytocin a postpituitary hormone that stimulates uterine contraction after delivery of placenta, avoiding postpartum hemorrhage.

pasteurized the partial sterilization of a fluid by heating it at 144° to 149°F., which destroys certain organisms and undesirable bacteria that could produce disease, without destroying the chemical composition of the fluid.
pathological due to a disease.
pellagra a deficiency disease cuased by improper diet and characterized by skin lesions, gastrointestinal disturbances, and nervousness.
peristalsis rhythmic contractions of the alimentary canal.
physiologist one versed in the study of the functions of the organs of the body.
plasma the liquid part of the lymph and blood.

quacks those who pretend a knowledge they do not possess.

radiation the discharge of rays in all directions from a common center.

seborrheic afflicted with abnormal discharge of sebum from the glands of the skin.
senile physiologic deterioration accompanying the aging process, especially loss of mental faculties in old age.
specific anything especially adapted to a certain purpose.
structural pertaining to structure rather than another aspect.
subclinical pertaining to the period of time before appearance of typical symptoms of a disease.
supplement a nutrient that is added to supply that which is lacking in a product or to reinforce it.
synthesize the process of building a product from separated elements.

tissue a collection of similar cells and fibers that form structural material in the body.
toxemia distribution through the body of poisonous products of bacteria that grow in a focal site.
toxic poisonous.

urea constituent of urine and the final product of protein metabolism in the body.

viscera internal organs, especially the abdominal.

Diet therapy

adequate sufficient for specific requirements.
allergen any substance causing allergic symptoms.
amino acids the "building blocks" of protein.
anorexia loss of appetite.

bland diet meal plan in which all food that causes chemical, mechanical, or thermal irritation is avoided.
bulk large volume.

cardiovascular pertaining to the heart and blood vessels.
cirrhosis a chronic, progressive disease of the liver, essentially inflammatory.
constituents component parts.
corpuscle a blood cell.
cystic duct the duct of the gallbladder that unites with the hepatic duct from the liver to form the common bile duct.

defecation evacuation of the bowels.
desensitize to lessen or irradicate sensitivity to a product.
diverticulitis inflammation of one or more diverticula in the colon, causing stagnation of feces in the little distended sacs.

edema a condition in which excess fluids form within the body.
elimination excretion of waste products from the body by the skin, kidneys, and intestines.
erythrocytes red blood cells.
extracellular outside of and surrounding the cell.

fibrinogen a soluble protein in the blood plasma that is essential in the clotting of blood.

gastrointestinal pertaining to the stomach and intestines.
glomerulus a tuft of capillary loops projecting into the inside of renal capsule.

hemicellulose a substance that increases bulk in the stool and promotes regular evacuation from the bowels.
hepatic pertaining to the liver.
hepatic duct the canal that receives bile from the liver and unites with the cystic duct to form the common bile duct.
hypersensitivity excessively sensitive.
hyperthyroidism a condition caused by excessive secretion of the thyroid glands.
hypoglycemia pertaining to deficiency of sugar in the blood.

inflammation a response to an injury to the tissues.
inhibit to hold in check or restrain.
inorganic composed of inanimate matter.
insulin a protein hormone of the internal secretion of the islands of Langerhans in the pancreas that controls the level of blood sugar.
intracellular within a cell.
intravenous within or into a vein.

jaundice yellowness of the skin due to bile pigments in the blood.

kilogram (kg.) 1,000 grams.

lesion an injury or wound.

leukocytes white blood corpuscles.
liter 1.056 quarts.

macrocytes red blood corpuscles larger than normal.
microorganism a minute living organism not perceptible to the naked eye.
milliliter (ml.) $1/1000$ of a liter.
millimeter $1/1000$ of a meter.
misnomer an incorrect designation.
monosaccharide a sugar that cannot be separated into smaller units.
mucous membrane the membrane lining passages and cavities, which secrete mucus.

nephrosis a condition in which there are degenerative changes in the kidneys without
    the occurrence of inflammation.
neurological pertaining to the study of nervous diseases.
neurotic an emotionally unstable individual.

obesity an abnormal condition due to excessive deposits of fat in the body.
occlusion the closing of a passage.
osmotic pressure pressure causing the passage of solutions of different concentrations
    through a membrane.

parenterally either within or into a vein or subcutaneously (beneath the skin).
pericarditis inflammation of the membranous sac enclosing the heart.
peritoneal cavity the region containing all the abdominal organs except the kidney.
plasma the liquid part of the blood in which the corpuscles and platelets float.
platelet a small circular or oval disk that is found in the blood and takes part in the coagu-
    lation of the blood.
polyuria excessive secretion and discharge of urine.
prothrombin substance present in the blood plasma and essential for the clotting of
    blood.
psychotherapy any mental method of treating disease, especially nervous disorders.

regeneration repair, regrowth, or restoration of a part.
residue that which remains after roughage is removed.
retina the sensitive membrane of the eye that receives the image formed by the lens,
    and that is connected with the brain by the optic nerve.
roughage the indigestible fibers of fruits and vegetables.

satiety satisfaction.
spleen an organ that disintegrates the red blood cell when its usefulness is ended and
    sets free the iron contained in the cell.

therapeutic nutrition that branch of nutrition concerned with the treatment of disease.
thermal pertaining to heat.

uremia the retention in the blood of urinary constituents due to failure of the kidneys to
    excrete them.
ureter one of the two tubes carrying urine from the kidney to the bladder.

varices enlarged, twisted veins.
vascular pertaining to or composed of blood vessels.

Index